A Life in Neurosurgery

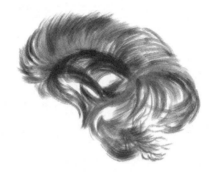

A Life in Neurosurgery

From Air Studies to Genomic Medicine

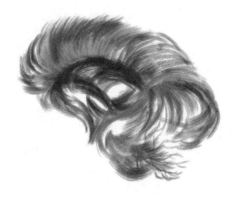

Meeting the Twenty-First Century
Challenge in Neuroscience

Patrick Elwood

Library of Congress Cataloging-in-Publication Data
Elwood, Patrick W., author

A Life in Neurosurgery; From Air Studies to
Genomic Medicine; Meeting the Twenty-First
Century Challenge in Neuroscience by Patrick
Elwood

ISBN 978-0-9975378-0-2

Neurosurgery 2 Neurological Care 3. Population
Health 4. Medical Education

Front Cover: Scott Barrows, Jump Trading Simulation and Education Center
Back Cover photo: Jim Carlson/OSF HealthCare

Published by White Oak Court Press
Peoria, Illinois

For John Shroyer, my chemistry professor
who changed the course of my life

Table of Contents

Table of Contents

Table of Contents

Table of Contents

PART II
MEETING THE TWENTY-FIRST CENTURY CHALLENGE IN NEUROSCIENCE

Table of Contents

Introduction

An Unplanned Journey

It was raining heavily Saturday afternoon as I sought cover in Logan Brothers Bookstore on West Harrison Street. The old-fashioned medical bookstore next to Cook County Hospital in Chicago's west side, was a favorite haven on cold wintery weekends, during medical school in 1955. Wilder Penfield's *Epilepsy and Functional Anatomy of the Human Brain* lay in the front of the new books table. My life in neuroscience began that afternoon. Penfield was an American Rhodes Scholar who founded the Montreal Neurological Institute with the support of the Rockefeller Foundation. He described work on treating epilepsy patients with brain surgery, while they were awake, the most exciting medical work I ever read. I finished the book that rainy weekend, and the direction of my life changed.

Sixty years later, I began a memoir for my children, Katherine, Eric, and John and their children so they might know what transpired while they were growing up in the family home on Moss Avenue in Peoria, Illinois in the '60s. As this book evolved, I realized I lived through much of the development of neurology, neurological surgery, and neuroradiology as specialties. Participating in the creation of a medical school, neurology and neurosurgery residency programs, and a neurological center in a

1

non-metropolitan setting were memorable opportunities.

My life in neurosurgery has been a series of transitions in primary interest and commitment each decade. In recent years, my major interest has been neurological care for the next half-century. Americans are living into their '80s and illness of the brain and nervous system are an overwhelming twenty-first century medical challenge. This book, perhaps a " memoir of the future", is as much about what is to come as what has been; how will society cope with caring for the aging brain and spine? These memories of how far we have come give me optimism for the future and a sense of urgency.

When I first considered a career, neurological care was done in metropolitan centers; New York, Chicago, Toronto, Montreal, London, and Paris. I lived in a small Midwestern city surrounded by miles of corn and soybeans with a limited population to support a neurological program. The decentralization of American medical specialty care began in the '60s as specialists migrated to small cities and I was part of that process. My initial career concerned individual patients; later, I struggled with providing complex neurological care to people distant from large population centers. I will describe this evolution in my interests and responsibilities over a career.

I grew up in the country and attended a two-room grade school and this journey has been an exercise in serendipity. As I began this book, I was reading *Unplanned Journey, From Moss Side to Eden* by Alcon Copisarow, a multi-talented English scientist and advisor to the UK government who describes an exceptional career, going from one role to another, seemingly without plan. (1) On a smaller scale, I also had multiple opportunities present through no planning or action on my part. This book is an effort to describe this unplanned path from a simpler America to one filled with challenge and opportunity.

I have worked with wonderful colleagues, some named in

this book and many not mentioned. The patient experiences all happened essentially as described with the names and details changed to protect patient and their family privacy. At times descriptions are excessively clinical and technical for some readers, and simplistic for clinical colleagues. I struggled with this problem without resolution and can only apologize for dull and heavy writing. In the process of writing about long ago events, opportunities overlooked and missteps became clear, prompting a great deal of analysis of needed change and improvement. At times, I digress to impart this wisdom to the reader utilizing my invaluable hindsight.

The half-century brought momentous change in the organization of society, medical care, medical education, and the expectations of society, an "unplanned journey". Life expectancy has increased, generally individuals age better, and these advances require a disruptive change in medical care. When I began practice, medical care was relatively simple, often inadequate, and an insignificant part of the national budget. In 1960 health care represented five percent of the Gross Domestic Product (GDP) or $27.4 billion and today it is $2.9 trillion with 18 percent of GDP. We have wonderful opportunities to better serve as a result of new technology and understanding of disease mechanisms.

In this process, medicine is often viewed as having lost much of its humanity, perceived as self-serving, and at times seems to have lost its way as a profession. I am concerned my colleagues lack a sense of urgency for applying technology to ease the burden of neurological illness. As this book evolved, my interests changed from recalling the past to critically looking at current work, and speculation regarding the change needed to be a more responsive profession better serving the American people. Looking at the process from outside, medical care seems dysfunctional. Building a system of medical care that will serve the American people is a complex challenge, and neurological care has its unique puzzles.

Providing what people really need is difficult, or we would be doing it. Some of the characteristics of neurological illness compound the difficulties experienced in general medicine. The challenges and opportunities in each neurological specialty are discussed in Chapter 8, relating the problems to my experience at the Illinois Neurological Institute (INI) in the past decade. A portion of this chapter particularly contains terms that hopefully are partially clarified in the limited glossary. In some respects, this book is also a memoir of the INI and the struggle to develop a Midwestern neurological center. The INI was formed primarily as an educational support system in 1991, and with OSF Health-Care developed as a hospital within a hospital in 2001. The INI assumed responsibility for the Neuroscience Service Line within all of OSF HealthCare in 2008. Hopefully, these ruminations and experiences will be of value to those charged with improving neurological care.

Neurological illness is manifest in many ways, with numerous common problems and some rare debilitating illnesses occurring in all age groups, creating a challenge to deliver comprehensive care. Back pain is virtually universal; muscular dystrophies are extremely rare. Common clinical problems are often managed by primary care physicians with occasional consultation; rare illnesses are only recognized and managed by a subspecialty neurologist. Illnesses, such as low back pain, are chronic and gradual in onset and immediate decisions are not necessary. On the other hand, an acute epidural hematoma (blood clot over the surface of the brain caused by an injury) in a five-year-old child must be managed within 30-40 minutes to prevent lifetime disability or death. Ischemic stroke, a plugged brain blood vessel, one of the common conditions managed by neurologists has a relatively narrow 4.5-hour treatment window requiring early recognition by patient and family. Great progress has been made in stroke treatment after presentation within the treatment window, but essentially no improvement has occurred in patient's timely arrival for care. This remains a challenge and a failure in "population medicine". The behavior of patients and their families remains unchanged, and the delay in seeking care after stroke is unexplained.

Chronic neurological diseases produce life-altering disability affecting patient and family livelihood and social structure. Illnesses are responsible for prolonged unemployment, loss of insurance, and loss of critical support mechanisms. Management requires the creation of multi-disciplinary teams of social workers, care providers, psychologists, and others, each generating recruitment and funding challenges. Assembling and financing the teams is a difficult social challenge. Immediate work in population health needs to address the extensive burden of neurological illness.

A critical shortage of neurological manpower compounds the problem, particularly severe in "flyover" small-town America. A shortfall of various neurological specialists is projected to steadily worsen over the next decade. (2) A current shortage of adult neurology specialists is projected to worsen to 20 percent by 2020. The average wait time for a new patient in 2010 was 28.1 days and had increased to 34.8 days in 2012 vs. 15.5 days in cardiology. Although enrollment in neurology residencies has recently improved, residency positions have been consistently underfilled in the past two decades. General neurologists have become rare, as residents almost universally take specialty fellowships. During the same period, reimbursement trends have driven neurologists to pursue interventional office practice and to leave hospital acute neurology practice associated with on-call responsibilities.

Child neurology presents an even greater challenge with a long training period (2 years pediatrics, 3 years of pediatric neurology), and patient visits that are long and inadequately reimbursed. Thirty-nine percent of children's hospitals in 2012 reported vacancies requiring over twelve months to fill. The new patient waiting time for children's neurology is often in excess of 45 days. Although there are only 72 training programs, some positions remain unfilled, perhaps because of problems associated with specialty reimbursement. Brain function is fascinating, neurological conditions are the subject of extremely rewarding research, clinical neuroscience is a wonderful way to spend your life. As neurological educators, we continue to do an extremely poor job of demonstrating the wonder to high school, university, and medical students.

Internists, family physicians, and pediatricians in most large systems have become less involved with the care of neurological illness, because of time demands and productivity compensation models that encourage early specialist referral. During the same period in the past two decades, neurological education as part of the residency program in medicine or pediatrics has virtually disappeared resulting in a rising group of primary care physicians ill-equipped to evaluate neurological problems. "Neurophobia" does exist in American medical education. (3) Medical students and general physicians believe neurological illness is mysterious and impenetrable. The indirect effect of the physician compensation model is to increase the demand for adult and pediatric neurological consultation and increase imaging and testing. Unfortunately the health care system business model for the internal medicine physician does not reward spending time with the patient in careful examination and thoughtful analysis.

Although the shortage of neurosurgeons is less acute, they are poorly distributed in the United States. Neurosurgical emergency room coverage is often difficult to achieve, requiring more neurosurgeons than the region can support based on the regional requirement for elective neurosurgical care. A neurosurgeon must be busy enough with his/her procedures to achieve economic stability and have the numbers of cases and variety to maintain competence throughout a long career. More neurosurgeons are joining large subspecialty groups challenging the service to less urban areas.

Geographic challenges in neurological care exist in rural America. Outside of large metropolitan areas, travel distance impairs care. Multiple sclerosis patients with movement limiting disability have to travel great distances to benefit from the current progress in neuro-immunology. There are areas in rural America that cannot provide adequate stroke care. Some small and midsized hospitals have neither the immediate demand nor the catchment to mount an acceptable care program for emergency neurosurgery or the neurological subspecialties. The result is less than optimum care for patients in rural America.

Multiple remedies have been applied; often specialists travel to outlying clinics, an ineffective utilization of their time and skill. The patient often requires the complex spectrum of care offered in a multi-disciplinary specialty clinic. In a multi-hospital medical care system, a well-developed portfolio of care should address caring for patients with complex needs over a rural geography while being cost-effective. With care protocols, specialty organization, and Tele-Neurology technology we will provide excellent care in rural areas with less travel by disabled patients and their families.

This book will seem a hodgepodge to the reader, wandering from a specific anecdotal clinical problem to the development of programs or speculation regarding future improvement. This reflects the reality of my life spent in clinical medicine while developing educational programs and clinical facilities. Medical emergencies push other matters away for the moment in a career combining clinical neurosurgery and leadership of neuroscience programs. A physician in an administrative role who remains clinically active retains a sense of reality that validates their contribution to the healthcare system. We straddle the administrative and clinical world to provide the care Americans need. This book describes my half-century of work in both worlds and the preparation needed to cope with the challenges of the remainder of the century. The technology and the resources exist today to care for the people in the United States coping with neurological illness; execution is our challenge.

Part I

A Life in Neurosurgery

Chapter 1

Peoria Early Days
1932-1952

*The beginning is the most important part
of the work*

—Plato

The Family Arrives in Peoria

The Elwood family arrived in Peoria early in the century, when John Elwood moved from Marshalltown, Iowa, to Peoria in 1924 to be a machinist at the newly formed Caterpillar Tractor Company. John left high school after the tenth grade to train as a machinist in the machine shops of the Minneapolis and St. Louis Railroad in Marshalltown. His father, Patrick Edward Elwood was a freight conductor on the M & St. L. Holt Tractor Company manufactured in Peoria and Stockton, California, and competed with the Best Gas Tractor Company of California. The two firms merged forming Caterpillar Tractor Company, based in Peoria, assuring stable employment. John Elwood arrived at the right time and soon became the night supervisor of the company. (1)

Mother, Mary Hamblin moved from Ramsay, a small town in southern Illinois, for an opportunity with a clothing manufacturer to create complex tailoring and a line of quality clothing. In that era, regional products were produced by relatively small local companies. Chic manufacturing in Peoria developed the Princess Peggy Brand, one of the large manufacturers of women's and girl's clothing. John and Mary married, and I was born September 11, 1932, with the country mired in the Great Depression. Throughout the depression, Caterpillar worked at least 4 days a week, supplying tractors for the Russian farm collectivization and other export markets, and the Elwood's were spared the hardships of the depression.

When I was three years old, my twin sisters, LuAnn and JoAnn were born. Dad moved us to a rural area, west of Peoria, to an acre of land containing a large vegetable garden, pear orchard, chicken yard, and small vineyard. This small piece of ground allowed us to grow virtually everything we ate. Dad was probably the first of the "hippies" growing what we ate and living simply in the country. He read the gardening catalogs avidly, finding things to grow, even attempting to grow peanuts in Central Illinois. Mom canned all the vegetables, and we filled a large root cellar. My job was fighting weeds and bugs in this early "organic" food production.

At the same time Dad was pursuing this self-sufficiency program, he was participating in the rapid development of a successful Caterpillar Tractor Company, soon becoming manager of the Tractor Division. His brother Randall moved from Iowa to join the company, ultimately becoming the manager of the Engine Division. Family conversations were heavy with engineering and manufacturing. Dad had my engineering school selected when I was six.

Our move to the country provided the opportunity to attend Pleasant Valley School, a two-room school about a mile from our home on Old Farmington Road, a two-lane gravel road. Pleasant Valley School had a substantial effect on my development. The school had 4 grades in each room, with about 8 students in each grade and a teacher for the "little room" and the "big room". The teacher in the "big room" had charge of the library and the paddle that was employed for the discipline of the larger boys. Since the next higher grade was in a row immediately to our left, it allowed one to advance as one's interest and drive allowed, an unintentionally progressive education program.

At the end of the third grade, I had completed the fourth grade work, so I left for the "big room" skipping the fourth grade. The "big room" gave access to a modest school library, and an opportunity to read as many books as I wanted. I lacked athletic ability, was the smallest boy in the grade, and hence, was never chosen for games. I found fun in reading, school work, and caring for my garden and chickens. At one point, by getting up very early, I was reading a book every 1-2 days with a goal to read all of the books in the library. Father allowed me to pick the pears and sell them for a dollar a bushel, developing work habits and time management.

The children at Pleasant Valley lacked great aspirations and a sense of academic competition. The people of the community were concerned with getting the day's work done rather than "career building". I was experiencing an idyllic childhood free of stress and the high expectations of today's suburbia. "Tiger mothers" were for another era.

Dad purchased a 120-acre farm near Fairview in 1932 in the depths of the depression, paying $125A, then about the highest price paid for farm land with outstandingly fertile soil. Dad arranged for George Overcash to farm the land and live there. In addition to corn, oats, and wheat, we raised a few pigs and cattle that supplied meat for our family and Mr. Overcash's family. Dad took me to the farm often, and I became attached to the young pigs and cows. Rural electricity was rare at that time, and the radio was served by a windmill charged battery, an early application of wind power. Kerosene lamps provided light at night in the house and barn. Mr. Overcash farmed with horses, and later purchased a tractor. Corn was picked by hand, and the picking took most of the winter and was hard painful work. Although one and two-row corn pickers were developed in the '20s, we were concerned that they left corn in the field, so Dad delayed the purchase of a corn picker until I was six years old.

The need to consistently work while going to school had a positive effect on my ability to pursue multiple tasks with enthusiasm and get things done. I recall unpleasant tasks, particularly harvesting alfalfa hay, being covered with small pieces of the drying hay while sweating, itching, and developing sunburn. Later the practice of medicine seemed easy in comparison!

I recall the concern regarding the declaration of war at the bombing of Pearl Harbor in December 1941. Dad was not drafted because he was 41 and was the manager of the Tractor Division at Caterpillar, considered an essential war function. Because of his work, he was given a "B" sticker for gasoline, allowing four gallons per week. This gave us some mobility and the ability to get to the farm. No private automobiles were manufactured, so we kept our 1936 Plymouth running through the war and obtained a new Ford in 1949. Since we raised our food either at home or on the farm, we experienced little privation during the war. The *Peoria Journal* published a war map on the front page each day, showing the battle lines in Europe and I followed the course of the war daily. This provided an excellent grounding in rapidly changing European geography.

Our neighbor, who was a conscientious objector, worked at the United States Department of Agriculture Research Laboratory during the war. I believe he was working on the penicillin project toward the close of the war. The other neighbors were involved in combat, one in the Merchant Marine in the North Atlantic, one in the Marines in the South Pacific, and one in the land war in France and Germany. All returned without injury at the end of the war.

There was no high school in the country, so the Limestone Township school district paid tuition for high school in Peoria. There were three high schools in Peoria, with Peoria High School having the best academic program. I had transportation to Woodruff High in the north side, so I entered Woodruff at age 12. Although Mom and Dad clearly expected me to work hard and bring home excellent grades, they did not appreciate the differences in academic programs. I went from a school with 80 students to a school with 1,500, from the country to the city.

Woodruff High School, Off to the City

E.N. Woodruff High School was an inner city school without academic pretensions named after a former mayor famous for maintaining gambling and prostitution in Peoria. There were some wonderful teachers that made a difference. My algebra teacher, Mildred Martin, aspired to help each student achieve their potential. Work was assigned each day and graded carefully. If not to her satisfaction, we returned for remediation at the end of the day. Miss Martin had high standards, there were students there every night. This experience of expecting excellence had an extraordinary, lasting effect on my life, convincing me that goals were achievable with hard work.

In the third year, American Government was required, taught by Andrew Heflin with enthusiasm, high expectations, with extra references, writing, and essays. This program, for the first time, exposed me to developing a reading program and writing lengthy essays. Mr. Heflin introduced me to a world of high expectations. In the final year, Miss Martin's sister, Dorthea Martin taught English literature and rhetoric. She assigned an essay each week that was edited heavily with a red pencil, and rewritten until the red pencil was no longer necessary. Virtually everyone finishing her rhetoric class could write a competent English essay, an astonishing feat of pedagogy.

Despite science being taught without the Martin sisters enthusiasm, I developed an interest in chemistry and felt I might become a scientist, perhaps a chemist. Mom insisted on typing, resulting in my enrollment in a class with 29 girls, all faster typists. With the advent of computers, her insistence seemed providential, but the experience was humbling.

Physical education was required and was a recurring torture with my lack of athletic ability and interest. In wrestling, even though I was in the lightweight class, I was invariably "pinned" almost instantly. The experience seemed pointless and of little value. As a result of the grades in typing and physical education, my academic averages were sound but not outstanding resulting in my graduating 17th in the class.

The SAT and ACT examinations, now the bane of student existence, did not trouble us in 1948. The first SAT was created in 1952 and half a million students took the test by 1957. The ACT was created in 1959 and heavily utilized in the Midwest, but we were blissfully unstressed by testing at Woodruff 1945. We lacked a system of academic counseling in preparation for University. Most students graduating from Woodruff High School went to work for Caterpillar; some went to the hospital nursing schools in Peoria, and a few attended Bradley University, the state teachers colleges, or the University of Illinois and some enlisted in the military. I do not recall any classmates considering travel out of the state to attend University, nor do I recall speaking with anyone with aspirations for professional school.

I suspect that there were some students at Peoria High School, the more academic high school across town, who aspired to distant university admission, as mentored by family or faculty. The Woodruff faculty did not make the students aware of the great world of opportunity, and perhaps they were unaware of a greater academic world. I missed mentoring and did not even realize it existed. A generation later, I had an opportunity to revisit the role of the public schools in Peoria with my children.

As the city moved north, and Richwoods High School was built, attendance in the inner city schools decreased, and eventually, Woodruff High School was closed in 2010, with a portion of the facilities utilized for vocational education.

Although I had several inspiring teachers at Woodruff, this was the first experience of less than optimum mentoring subsequently repeated in University, Medical School and Neurosurgery Residency. One of the most important roles of education is an accurate assessment of student ability and encouragement to fully utilize that potential. I did not pursue mentoring and advice and this failing was shared by my classmates. This remains an important problem in inner-city schools where the counselors are a surrogate for parental guidance. In affluent suburbs, the mentoring function is less critical because the parents impart sophisticated knowledge and expectations.

This fundamental deficit at the primary and secondary school level is a factor in our societal problems of income inequality, massive underemployment, and crime. Children who know what can be accomplished and are encouraged often achieve at their ability level. Students in the inner city often are unaware of opportunities, and teachers sometimes assume that knowledge is unnecessary. Wasted lives and a loss to society are the result.

Over the years, as we developed the medical school and graduate programs, I had an opportunity to accept mentoring responsibilities. I have occasionally succeeded, but often failed as the result of lack of focus and timely recognition of the right moment. This is one of the greatest opportunities to introduce excitement in people's lives and prevent some of the societal problems created by apathy. I owe Miss Mildred Martin, Mr. Heflin, and Miss Dorthea Martin a great deal; they opened the world of high expectations and provided a challenge. I regret that my realization of this debt came too late for me to thank them. Avoid this mistake.

Hunts Drive-In, Economics 101

At 16, employment outside of home and farm was legal, and I obtained a job as a curb waiter at Hunts Drive-In, a Peoria institution. The Drive-In was at the base of Bradley Park, about three miles from home and I commuted by bicycle. A kitchen building was surrounded by a large parking lot that accommodated 90 cars in six concentric circles. It was unique in a world before the advent of "fast food". Mr. Hunt employed high school students from Peoria, paying 30 cents an hour, and allowing us to have food worth 60 cents for our dinner. We were allowed to keep the tips the customers gave us. My paycheck for a six-day week was $13.20. We worked seven hours 4 days a week and eight hours a day on the 2-day week end.

When a car drove in and parked, several of us raced to the car, the one arriving first took the order, and after the food was prepared brought it to the car. We took the tray away when they flashed their lights or honked to indicate they were finished and received our tip. Superb service was assured because so much of the income was generated by the tip, and Mr. Hunt had a draconian incentive plan. Each week, he posted the number of orders taken by each curb waiter. Usually, each week, the last one on the list lost his position, generating some turnover, but customers never waited for anything.

The night Mr. Hunt hired me, it was raining, things were slow, and we sat in his veranda office listening to the rain as he outlined his fundamental business philosophy to me. It was rather harsh, but clearly was a service-oriented philosophy that is just now being taught and encouraged in health care. In health care, it has taken us a century to propose "patient-centered care". We often execute poorly, certainly never as well as Mr. Hunt circa 1948.

Hunt's Drive-In is gone and generally people no longer eat in their automobiles, instead going through drive through or sitting down in a "Fast Food" chain. Mr. Hunt introduced me to meeting the customer's need early in my life. His service execution was simple and superb.

Away to College, Not Far

After finishing high school, neither Mom, Dad nor I gave much thought to college destination. Dad always thought I would be an engineer, but the career choice was mine. Although I had worked hard in high school, my academic record was undistinguished. I entered Bradley University in the fall of 1949, allowing me to live at home, commute, and experience little life change. No sense of adventure evident.

Although Bradley Hall and the Horology School were classic stone buildings, most of the campus buildings were WW II military surplus. The student body was a mixture of those fresh from high school and returning veterans on the GI Bill. In the late spring after starting college, the male students were called in and informed that they should consider joining the Air Force ROTC program. North Korean People's Army had poured across the 38th parallel on June 25, 1950. Students were at draft risk to serve in the Korean War. I became an air force ROTC cadet, with the intention to receive a commission and attend flying school after graduation.

I decided to do something in science, probably chemistry and pursued that with vigor. Organic chemistry changed my life direction. Dr. John Shroyer, Professor of Chemistry and Department Head, quizzed me in the laboratory each day pushing me to my limit. He showed me I was capable of sustained complex intellectual work and could be an excellent student. For the first time I worked at capacity, and it was exciting. Dr. Shroyer was the most stimulating mentor I experienced throughout my career.

I began to feel that I needed more contact with people than a laboratory career would provide, and considered medical school. Dr. Bhagat Singh was as demanding in physical chemistry as Dr. Shroyer had been, allowing me to satisfy the requirements for admission to the College of Medicine in three years. I lived the life of a commuting student, was not exposed to students from a wide geography and was the only one attending medical school from the Bradley class of 1953. My intellectual horizons had not been greatly expanded by the Bradley experience, but Shroyer and Singh convinced me that science was exciting, and I had the ability to do science. Bradley served me well.

I had little advice concerning medical school, and was unaware admission was difficult. I knew nothing about the MCAT, then in its infancy, only that I had to travel to Knox College in Galesburg for the examination. I simply sat the examination without preparation; Kaplan preparation courses were in the future. I applied to Washington University and the University of Illinois. Washington University offered a position almost immediately, but the tuition was over $1,000 a year. I refused the offered position and waited for admission to Illinois, which came later with a tuition of $365 a year. With this modest tuition, and work available, there was no accumulated debt from medical school, a freedom not experienced by our current students, who often graduate with a $100,000 to $200,000 debt burden.

After admission to medical school, I discussed enrollment with the Air Force Colonel. After some exploration, he indicated that the Air Force was willing to discharge me to attend medical school, ending my potential career as a fighter pilot in the Korean War, probably a fortunate decision. After three years of college, I would start medical school with the understanding that Bradley would award my degree with transfer credits from medical school at the end of the first year. I was awarded a B.S. degree with the class of 1953 but did not attend the graduation, fully occupied with challenges in the College of Medicine.

After a few less than impressive personal exposures to the world of medicine, Dad told me "medicine is an ideal career for a second-class mind". Engineering and manufacturing were best served with a first-class intellect. He did not attempt to dissuade or change my decision but clearly was disappointed.

Pabst Brewery: Labor Relations 101

Employment in industry was possible at 18, and my next summer job to earn tuition for medical school was in the Bottle House at Pabst Brewery in Peoria Heights. I spent most of my time feeding a large bottle washing machine with occasional rotations to other tasks. Although there were a few other college students working for the summer, most were regular employees. We worked twelve-hour shifts six days a week, two weeks during the day, then two weeks at night. The bottle house was filled with machinery, the noise was ear shattering, and protection was unavailable. The first week, my ears rang for one to two hours after leaving work. I was concerned that this noise would last forever. I seemed to gradually adapt and the ringing stopped. OSHA years later attacked this problem with required worker hearing protection.

This was my first exposure to people that drank throughout the day. We had a short break every two hours, and most employees drank beer and had a snack, thus a significant amount of beer was consumed in the course of a day. It was available in large ice-filled tubs throughout the plant but officially one was not allowed to drink while at a machine. Most employees knew their job well, and it could often be accomplished with relatively little work.

I was introduced to the reality of labor relations rather early in the course of my Pabst career. Assigned to clean up a bottling line, I attacked the problem with vigor, accomplishing the project in 6 hours. I later learned bottle line clean up ordinarily was a two day two man job. Suspension by the union followed with instructions to report to the business agent of the Brewery and Distillery Workers Union downtown the next day. He informed me I had caused problems with work expectations in the Bottle House. He would reinstate me, allowing me to work, if I promised that under no circumstances would I again work hard while employed at Pabst. An assurance was given, I simply had misunderstood, and was used to working on the farm. He reissued my temporary union membership card, and I was back to work. The regular union members were paid $1.77 per hour and the temporary permit holders were paid $1.43 per hour. Income from the long days met the tuition payments quite well. After two years, my brewery career was finished, without regret. The experience was of great value, providing me with a better understanding of the work and stress experienced by my future patients.

Chapter 2

Medicine Beginnings
1952-1957

Being Irish, he had an abiding sense of tragedy which
sustained him through temporary periods of joy

—W. B. Yeats

Four Years in Chicago's West Side

The Rock Island Rocket took me to Chicago, and the "L" took me from the LaSalle Street Station to the medical center. The ghetto and the industry of the south side along the railway was a discouraging introduction to Chicago on a grey September day. The University of Illinois, Cook County Hospital, and the Presbyterian Hospital were an urban island surrounded by west side ghetto with poverty and crime.

University housing on the west side was unavailable for students. Most of the non-commuting students lived in one of four medical fraternity houses along Ashland Avenue. A "rush" was conducted immediately before the semester began, allocating students to various fraternities. The "rush" was a four day period of beer consumption, and since that was not my forte, I failed to do well, matching with the "Phi Bete" house, the least popular fraternity associated with the poorest scholarship. "Phi Rho" had the best students and "Nu Sig" had most of the "important people".

I was assigned a double room with a rather unusual roommate who was remarkably bright, studied very little, and spent the evenings playing the violin and cutting hair in our room, making concentration and study difficult. The second year, a tiny room next to the dormitory sleeping room on the third floor was available offering solitude at a price. In a former life, it was a closet so it lacked a radiator. I spent the next three years in that room, always able to concentrate but often wearing an overcoat and gloves.

During the two basic science years, we had some sort of examination weekly that provided recurrent stress. A comprehensive examination occurred at the end of the second year. Usually after that examination, 20 to 30 students were asked to leave because of poor performance and were replaced by transfer students from the two-year medical schools in North and South Dakota. This rather unenlightened educational philosophy did encourage students to study but created fear and diminished respect for the Alma Mater. We envied the students downtown at Northwestern because they appeared to have virtually assured graduation after admission.

Biochemistry was the first year course that often led to a request to leave the college, and the first examination was a dreaded event. Walking back to the Phi Bete House on Ashland Avenue after the test, discussion with other students revealed to my consternation that my answers differed from my classmates. A number of the students were Chicagoans from "The Pier". Navy Pier had been opened as a branch campus of the University of Illinois after the War and was full of ultracompetitive pre-meds from the Chicago metropolitan area. Most attended the University of Illinois College of Medicine. The men from the Pier seemed to exude self-confidence in contrast to the country boys from down-state. After hearing their comments, I was convinced that this was probably my last month in medical school. On returning the next week, I found that I had received the only 100 grade and my answers were correct. I might last the semester.

We spent every afternoon in the gross anatomy dissection lab working on our cadaver with three partners. The class was alpha-betized in an impersonal fashion, so I worked with Ellis, England, and Etchyson. There were four large rooms interconnected in the seventh-floor anatomy laboratory. At the end of the semester, there was both a written and practical examination just before the semester break. On return after Christmas break, the anatomy professor walked around the laboratory and "tapped on the shoulder" those who had done poorly. They were invited to meet with the dean. On the first day back, Professor Zimmerman came by and tapped me. I immediately assumed that my stay in medical school was almost over. He returned late that morning and in his

German accent, told me I had the highest score in the class, and he felt I was an outstanding anatomist! At this point, I began to think I might get through this whole process and graduate.

It was not a collegial way to conduct the education of physicians. No one mentored like Dr. Shroyer that first year. The final part of the year we were taught neuroanatomy by Gerhardt von Bonin, a famous German neuroanatomist who lectured in a rather absent-minded fashion. He repeatedly pointed out that actually little was known about human function, the physiological knowledge was virtually entirely based on animal work. He walked about the front of the room in decrepit grey carpet slippers, seemed disorganized and was an unpopular professor. The students appreciated certainty and organization; the unknown and speculation seemed a waste of time. I enjoyed von Bonin's skepticism. Neuroanatomy and brain function was fascinating and for the first time, I felt that something in neuroscience might be a career.

The second year was even more packed and almost an inhuman experience with lectures and labs all day and several examinations each week. Pathology was the major course of the year and I attacked it with vigor. I read *Anderson's Pathology*, called "Big A", while many of my classmates utilized the synopsis version "Little A". Dr. Cecil Krakow, a Canadian kidney investigator gave innumerable lectures and had an uncanny skill of finding sleeping medical students with his pencil searchlight. Pharmacology was the other major course of the year and seemed an introduction to real clinical medicine at last. Goodman and Gilman *The Pharmacological Basis of Therapeutics* was a massive tome that became my temporary bible.

Dr. Percival Bailey, who had collaborated with Harvey Cushing as a neuropathologist and neurosurgeon taught neuropathology and did "brain cutting". He wrote a pioneering book on the histology and origin of the glioma series of brain tumors. He spent a great deal of time at La Pitie sal Petriere, the ancient neurological hospital in Paris and knew Babinski, one of the fathers of French neurology in Paris. Dr. Bailey was a fluent Francophone and wore a beret. His impressive scholarship reinforced my interest in neuroscience created by the neuroanatomy course.

The finale was the dreaded sophomore comprehensive examination, the challenge that stood between us and entering clinical medicine. Although not required, I also sat the national board examination. I felt it might be useful in future licensure. The national boards only achieved overwhelming importance in the residency selection process a few years later, after they became a required part of the graduation process in all US medical schools. Only a small portion of our class took the national board examination in the '50s.

There was a three-month break before the third clinical year, and I spent this in the laboratories in the basement of the Illinois Neuropsychiatric Institute, because of my interest in brain function. A cohesive, creative group was working there at the time, Ralph Gerard in Neurophysiology, Fred Gibbs in EEG, Gerhard von Bonin in Neuroanatomy, and Alex Geiger in Neurochemistry. I spent three months with Dr. Geiger isolating the circulation of the cat's brain, perfusing it with a blood substitute, and studying the chemistry of the brain. Dr. Geiger at the time had a great interest in the biochemistry of schizophrenia, and I became interested in the disease that summer, convinced that the answer was in neurochemistry. I entered the third year committed to neuroscience.

The third year was devoted to required clinical clerkships: pediatrics, medicine, surgery, and obstetrics. Although there was a series of neurological lectures, a neuroscience clinical experience was not part of the curriculum. During the clerkship we clerks were part of the treatment team with residents and interns, observing and learning, but not making treatment decisions. We were the most junior member of the team, writing notes in the chart, and taking care of various errands. The surgery clerkship was a new experience, but I came away feeling the surgeons were not asking challenging questions, and the work often seemed routine. Both my chief resident and Dr. William Grove, the young attending surgeon on the B service were supportive and interested in the students, yet lacked a "sense of wonder" in surgery.

The junior medicine clerkship was at the Cook County Hospital, and my principal attending physician was obviously fascinated by medicine. I presented two cases in detail each week, with a review of the appropriate literature. He asked searching questions and challenged me to identify unanswered questions. The problems of internal medicine were my forte, and I decided professor of medicine was my career goal. I began to associate with a group that clearly felt surgeons were an intellectually deprived group. We eagerly awaited the arrival of the *New England Journal of Medicine* each week and the weekly Clinical Pathological Conference (CPC) offered in the *Journal*. All the history, physical, and laboratory results were provided and it was our task to make the diagnosis.

The last year involved more advanced clerkships in medicine and surgery and a few elective experiences. Encouragement to participate in resident and faculty research was unusual. The class largely was unaware of the important unanswered questions and challenges in medicine; we were missing much of the excitement.

Dr. Oldberg, the Professor and Head of Neurosurgery trained by Harvey Cushing, gave a series of Saturday morning lectures in Neurosurgery that were uncommon exercises in clarity and succinctness. The lecture always started exactly at 8:00 a.m. when the door was locked, thus ensuring no stragglers. I did a short elective on the neurosurgery service at the Neuropsychiatric Institute (NPI).

As described in the introduction, on a rainy late Friday afternoon, in the Logan Brothers Book Store on Harrison Street, I found the book *Epilepsy and Functional Anatomy of the Human Brain* by

29

Wilder Penfield. I read a bit, found it intriguing and bought the book. I read non-stop through the weekend, almost finishing the 600+ page book, and was ready to change from internal medicine to "brain surgery" by late Sunday night. Penfield described patient after patient that he operated upon, while the patient was awake, to treat their epilepsy, describing the effect of stimulating one area of the brain after another. He had formed a team with Herbert Jasper, an electoencephalographer and Brenda Milner, a neuropsychologist, and they were finding how the brain worked while treating epilepsy patients from around the world.

Penfield was an exceptional person, born in Washington State, attended Princeton, was a Rhodes Scholar, started medical school at Oxford, and finished at Johns Hopkins. He became a neurosurgeon in New York, and then moved to Montreal to build a neurological institute with a $1.2 million grant from the Rockefeller Foundation and additional funds from Montreal and the Province of Quebec. The Montreal Neurological Institute opened as a hospital attached to the Royal Victoria Hospital in 1934. Penfield intended to build a multi-specialty team that would improve fundamental understanding of brain function, a fresh concept at the time that won Rockefeller support. Unlike other clinicians of his day, he was unsatisfied with day to day surgical treatment; he was interested in building a team that would discover how the brain worked. Although I never met Dr. Penfield, he had a major influence on my career and my life and was the major impetus for entering neurosurgery.

I began to ask about "brain surgery" and was told that it was a very interesting field, but there were already 300 neurosurgeons in the country. The field was full and earning a living would be impossible. Although there were some outstanding neurologists and neurosurgeons on the faculty, there were no required neuroscience clerkships. The University of Illinois College of Medicine was not a "hotbed " of neuroscience. Back to reading the *New*

England Journal of Medicine cover to cover each week and solving the clinical pathological case; professor of medicine remained my plan.

I was fast nearing the end of my experience in Chicago's west side and had to find a place for the next year. I made an appointment to talk with Professor Dowling, Chairman of Medicine about my career. He told me to stay at the "R and E" (University of Illinois Research and Educational Hospital) and really did not discuss other alternatives. I indicated I would like to see another center, and he told me that if I went, I could not return. Professor Dowling did not outline a program for an academic career in medicine, nor did he recommend a mentor. I left feeling that the Chairman of Medicine did not entirely understand his role as a student mentor in the College of Medicine.

I graduated with "high honor", the only member of the class so designated, yet never felt entirely confident that I would graduate or do well during the entire four-year experience. Perhaps more troubling, advice and mentoring were not offered. I left disappointed in the function of the State University. Although a few professors seemed excited about their work, none advocated the development of research skills or provided mentoring regarding the spectrum of careers available in medicine. Clearly, if assertive, I would have sought and found mentorship, I contributed substantially to the problem. Several classmates found excellent research opportunities and independently found excellent career advice. At the time, I had little appreciation for the opportunities lost and only came to understand the responsibilities of faculty with later teaching experience. Years later, the opportunity to offer a different experience occurred as we built a new medical school and graduate program in Peoria. Experiences in the College of Medicine made me understand the critical role of the professor in demonstrating career possibilities and providing encouragement to students to achieve all that they are capable of doing, the "John

Shroyer" approach to professorship.

I felt that I would get a unique experience in a large city hospital associated with a medical school. This would involve the care of indigent patients and "real personal experience". I looked at the city-county hospitals in Chicago, Philadelphia, Detroit, Milwaukee, Minneapolis and Saint Paul. The city hospitals I visited had an important and respected role in society at the time. Medicare and Medicaid had yet to be enacted, and a large part of society was medically indigent and sought care without a bill. Most of the city hospitals were major teaching hospitals for an associated medical school and the training ground for their residents in specialty training.

Since Medicare funding for graduate education was not available, residents were paid small stipends, ranging from nothing to $50 per month. They were usually expected to live in the hospital and were provided meals and laundry. A teaching appointment in the hospital was an important and prestigious responsibility of the faculty, who often were unpaid voluntary attending physicians. The Cook County Hospital had a competitive examination for sought-after positions as a two-year intern. Virtually all of the hospitals had large wards of 20-50 beds, with a few small rooms for the sickest and the dying. The wards were often managed by a senior nurse who had years of practical experience and was a resource for junior house officers. Indigent patients received care that cost relatively little in large wards without amenities. Inexpensive generic medications and physicians who were volunteers or who were serving with minuscule salaries kept costs low. It was an imperfect system, but patients left without debt or bankruptcy.

The Minneapolis General Hospital (MGH) attracted me because it was associated with the University of Minnesota and had an excellent Medicine Department. The hospital was old and seemed clean. Good care was provided to patients in 20-bed wards. The October day I visited Minneapolis, it was snowing and the significance escaped me. I didn't realize winter would be extremely cold and long and that frostbite would be commonplace! The formal intern matching structure of today did not exist; an offer was extended, and I signed a contract providing a salary of $25 a month, a room, food and laundry. There was a charge of $3 per month to park my 1949 Studebaker in an outside lot. The car did not start in subzero weather from November till April. The next year was now secure.

Minneapolis General Hospital

I arrived in Minneapolis and was immediately paired with two interns that I would work with for 12 months; Dick Sloop from the University of Oregon and Gerry Weil from the University of Colorado. Dick felt that Oregon was heaven; he spent the year telling me that it was the only place to live in the United States. At the end of the year, he returned, trained in general surgery, and practiced the rest of his life in Salem, Oregon. Gerry was born in Vienna and left shortly after the Anschluss in 1938. His father was placed in a concentration camp, unexpectedly released, and the family fled Austria immediately. Gerry, despite that experience, in 1956 was one of the few people in Minneapolis with a Volkswagen "Beetle." Gerry returned to Colorado, trained in pathology and spent the rest of his life in Colorado.

This was a "rotating internship" that involved serving on 13 services over the course of a year, providing exposure to all of medicine in a medium size city hospital caring for the indigent of Minneapolis. At that time, most internships, especially on the East Coast, were "straight" surgery or medicine, but in the Midwest and West, particularly in city hospitals, a rotating year was still offered. The Minneapolis General Hospital was affiliated with the University of Minnesota Medical School and shared some graduate programs with the University while other programs were independent. I began the year committed to a career as an academic internist, intending to move to the University Hospital for my medicine residency.

The hospital had a 20-bed ward in each wing with a few semi-private and private rooms adjacent to the ward. The psychiatry, tuberculosis, and the neurology wards were in the Annex building. Single house officers lived in a unit adjacent to the medicine ward.

I began the year on the obstetrical service and performed nine deliveries the first night, an impressive introduction to "being a real doctor" with all of the responsibility. I met my future wife, Gladys Thomas, the first week on the obstetrical service. Gladys was the very efficient charge nurse on the unit and clearly had a much more extensive knowledge of obstetrics than I possessed. It was a busy time, I learned a great deal, but retained my intellectual disdain for obstetrics, experiencing nothing on the service to alter my opinion.

Our life on the medicine service was split between managing the ward and an outpatient clinic where we cared for a number of largely elderly patients experiencing multiple illnesses. It seemed that every patient had diabetes, hypertension, pulmonary disease, and heart failure with arthritis as well. Despite careful review of massive charts and real effort in management, none of my patients seemed to make the slightest improvement.

An elderly man who I had treated for heart failure with modest success returned with massively swollen ankles, indicating chronic heart failure. He insisted he was taking his medication faithfully and there had been no change in his activities. After a lengthy review, he did admit one change in his routine. He had begun having a sardine soda cracker sandwich each night! An added salt load each night had greatly worsened his congestive heart failure.

After my experience on the medicine service, with further thought, I decided I did not have the patience or aptitude for an internal medicine career. My patients were not improving! The search resumed for something that would better fit my desire for demonstrable patient improvement. Internal medicine in the theoretical was challenging and clearly attracted the smartest people in medicine. The patients, however, did not seem to dramatically recover under my care. Internal medicine was not simply making brilliant diagnoses! It required thoughtful work and much more patience than I possessed. I began to reconsider neurosurgery and talked with some people at the University of Minnesota, referred to as the "The U" in the twin cities. They were not as discouraging as my friends in Chicago. At the time, open-heart surgery was beginning at the University of Minnesota with Dr. Lilliehei and Dr. Varco and this seemed of some interest as well. Both fields seemed rather undeveloped and challenging.

We were now deep into Minnesota winter, two months on the emergency service was next. The MGH was rather unique because we provided the ambulance service for the city and the interns rode the ambulance. My experience occurred in January-February, and I had the opportunity to take my gloves off and care for accident victims in 20 degree below zero weather. I first saw the effect of frostbite on ears, with men coming in with massive swelling of their ears after exposure without a hat. The ambulance drivers all had a great deal of experience, and were often quite helpful to the young, inexperienced interns as we encountered recurring unique challenges.

This was an opportunity to see an entirely different social world. There were a number of single room residential "hotels" near downtown Minneapolis where men employed in the summer by railroads, construction, and other fields spent the winter. Alcohol was their solace during the dark, cold winter months. Delirium tremens was common and the MGH ambulance was called to provide paraldehyde as a sedative to hold them over and calm their hallucinations or to take them to the hospital. Frequently, the

manager of the establishment asked us to see four or five hallu-
cinating, agitated tenants, while we were there. One evening, I
went on a call to one of the hotels to find that one man had his ear
bitten off, and his attacker had a stab wound of the arm. The police
officer asked that I take both patients back in the same ambulance.
I declined, arranging a separate ambulance for each, avoiding the
role of peacemaker for these two combatants.

The ambulance service also provided a new view of the elderly
poor. Elderly women sometimes called because they were lonely
and depressed and the ambulance crew visit was helpful. Many
of the elderly lacked family in the Twin Cities, and they relied on
service from the MGH. Dealing with illness in patients, whilst in
their woefully inadequate home facility, was strikingly different
from the sterile hospital environment. Today, with the loss of these
services and the house call, younger physicians have less understanding of the reality of patient's lives.

The rotating internship provided an opportunity to be busy
and responsible in virtually every field of medicine in a short
time. This unique opportunity is no longer available in today's
more regimented world of graduate medical education. Surgery
was an exhausting experience in that we were on call two nights
out of three. We usually operated all night the first night and were
allowed to go to bed at midnight the second night unless the service
was swamped. Recognition of the risks of sleep deprivation was
in the distant future. Our responsibility was clear, we were the
only staff available to provide care. Many of the surgical residents
planned to return to their homes in the Dakotas', where they
would perform emergency orthopedic surgery, general surgery,
and gynecologic surgery. They were truly "general" surgeons and
often the only resource in their community.

The attending neurosurgeon, Dr. Harold Buckstein, visited
several times a week and saw patients with us. It seemed that he
never took his camel hair overcoat off as he made ward rounds,

and largely advised that "nothing could be done" with most of our patients. This sadly was an accurate indication of the state of neurosurgery in 1956. I did have a salvageable patient, however, who arrived while gradually losing consciousness. A skull x-ray demonstrated that the calcified pineal gland that is supposed to be in the middle of the brain was shifted laterally 10 mm. In that era, a "pineal shift" was considered a valuable indicator of a mass in the brain. Dr. Buckstein told the surgical resident to take the patient to surgery and place a burr hole on each side of the back of the head under local anesthesia. I promptly did that and drained a subdural hematoma that looked for all the world like old motor oil. While on the table, the patient began to awaken and swear prodigiously. When his incision was sutured, he was ready for a fight. Neurosurgery immediately seemed more therapeutic than internal medicine.

Time was slipping away. I was preoccupied, very busy and needed a plan for a job next year. I was undecided but inclined to pursue surgical work, perhaps neurosurgery or cardiac surgery. Dr. William Grove, the second man in the surgery department at the University of Illinois, had been very supportive in medical school and I reached out to him and visited Chicago. The surgical program, at that time, took three residents per year, and it was difficult to get one of those positions. Those entering the program were expected to complete the full four years of general surgery. Dr. Grove and Dr. Warren Cole, head of the surgery department, agreed to take me on as a fourth man in the program, calling me a senior surgical intern to distinguish me from my fellow three junior assistant surgical residents. I would work with William Marshall, Jackson Cagle, and Arthur Williamson the next year while finding my way into an appropriate career. I would have to leave at the end of the year.

During this period, Gladys was attending the University of Minnesota, playing a lot of golf, and working as an obstetrical nurse at MGH. We were occasionally canoeing on Lake Harriet or having an ice cream cone at the village by the U. I asked her to accompany me to Chicago and we became engaged. She took a position teaching pediatric nursing at the Children's Hospital of Cook County Hospital, arriving shortly after I settled into the surgical service. We were embarking on a move without a clear plan beyond the one-year appointment.

Polio Conquered

Jim Thorn, a 21- year-old construction worker, felt a little achy Wednesday, then Thursday awakened with his arms and legs feeling much worse. He decided to lie down, fell asleep for an hour and on awakening could not get out of bed because of profound arm and leg weakness. His mother called the Minneapolis General Hospital ambulance and he was brought to the emergency room. A spinal tap was done, the ER staff made a diagnosis of polio and admitted Jim to the 9th-floor infectious disease unit. I was the admitting intern, spending one month on the infectious disease service the summer I arrived in Minneapolis.

On Jim's arrival on the unit, he was having difficulty breathing and it was clear he had bulbar polio. The virus involved the centers responsible for his diaphragm function, and he also had some difficulty coughing. Working with my medicine resident, we placed him in a large tubular Drinker Respirator (called the Iron Lung) that breathed for him. The Drinker made a loud swishing sound as it alternately expanded his rib cage, and seemed to make him remarkably inaccessible to the staff caring for him. The nurses gave skin care, started IV's and other activities through small ports that gripped their arms so that the vacuum was not lost and the patient continued to breathe. Jim stabilized relatively well and tolerated being in the Drinker without a great deal of fear. During the month I was on the service his condition remained essentially the same. Fortunately, the disease did not advance after the second day. The following month, Jim gradually improved and was weaned out of the respirator and began a rehabilitation program.

During my month on service, we had two patients in Drinker respirators, and both continued to require respiratory support. Over time, fortunate patients gradually improved and regained the ability to breathe, and unfortunate patients either died of a lung infection or remained permanently in the respirator. Other patients with polio had paralysis of legs or arms in a rather haphazard fashion that again improved in an unpredictable fashion. Most Americans recall the effect of this illness on President Roosevelt, probably the most famous polio victim.

Almost every summer, an outbreak terrifying families occurred somewhere in the United States. Parents would not allow their children to swim, attend parties, or participate in group activities. Since the illness was poorly understood, why some were struck down and others escaped seemed a mystery holding the nation in its grip. Long afterward, it is hard to comprehend the recurring fear that fell over the land every summer.

Minneapolis was the home of the Sister Kenny Institute established to assist patients in the recovery from paralysis with an elaborate program of hot packs and therapy. Patients came from around the United States for treatment at this center. Elizabeth Kenny was an Australian army nurse who was addressed as "Sister" as nurses were in Commonwealth countries. She treated her first polio case in 1911 with moist hot packs and stretching with muscle "re-education." She came to the United States in 1940 and established the Sister Kenny Institute in 1942, which soon developed into a 100- bed hospital.

Dr. Jonas Salk developed an inactivated polio virus vaccine using HeLa cells. It was first tested in 1952 and approved in 1955 after the largest medical experiment in history, the Francis Field

Trial. (1) During the trial, 440,000 children received the vaccine, 210,000 received a placebo, and 1.2 million in the control group received no vaccine. The results were announced April 12, 1955. After school began that fall, all of the house officers at the Minneapolis General Hospital that could be spared were dispatched to the public schools with MGH nurses, and every child in Minneapolis was given the Salk vaccine in a single day.

Poliomyelitis was essentially eradicated in Minneapolis that day, a profound demonstration of the world-changing effect of basic research applied to medicine. An illness that had terrified parents every summer for years was conquered seemingly overnight! Millions of dollars were expended for care of poliomyelitis victims over many years with limited benefit and much human suffering and disability. Fundamental research eradicated the disease. A significant part of orthopedic surgery in children was devoted to reconstructive efforts with fusions and tendon transfers to improve the function of paralyzed limbs. In a short time, numerous orthopedic procedures and associated infrastructure became unnecessary. The vaccine had a significant effect on pediatric orthopedic surgery practice.

This personal experience impressed me with the astounding potential for disruptive change created by basic research. Our congressmen and medical leadership seem to have forgotten this when making funding allocation decisions today. Importance has been placed on immediate "practical" results, and funding is being changed to "patient-centered outcomes research". Although outcomes have been a neglected area needing the attention now received, it must not be developed by diminishing National Institute of Neurological Disorders and Stroke (NINDS) funding for fundamental research, such as work that yielded the Salk and Sabin vaccine. Funding by the National Institutes of Health (NIH) and NINDS has diminished to the point that a relatively small portion of research grant proposals receive funding. A career in neuroscience research is precarious indeed, seemingly dependent on the Congressional mood. The Polio saga is an important reminder of the immense value of basic science research in disease mechanisms that seemingly has no immediate practical value, but has potential for disruptive change.

An oral vaccine was subsequently developed by Albert Sabin using an attenuated poliovirus, with trials beginning in 1957, and vaccine approved and placed in use in 1962. With availability of a vaccine, the worldwide incidence of polio soon dropped to about 220 cases. The story is a vivid reminder of the effectiveness of appropriate vaccination. The developing reluctance of parents regarding vaccination could create a danger that poliomyelitis will resurface as a childhood scourge. After a frightening disease such as polio or measles has been virtually eliminated and the associated public terror dissipated, the critical importance of universal vaccination in disease control is forgotten.

The Sister Kenny Institute merged with the Courage Center to form the Courage Kenny Rehabilitation Institute, part of Allina Health providing a comprehensive rehabilitation program. Their journey is a demonstration of change in mission with the eradication of the fundamental reason for the original creation of the institution.

Back to Chicago to Find My Way

I began work July 1, after driving overnight from Minneapolis in the old Studebaker. I fell asleep at the wheel just south of the Wisconsin border but awakened without an accident. An early personal experience with sleep deprivation. I was provided a room on the 8th-floor at the Neuropsychiatric Institute and was available in the hospital much of the time.

There were three surgical patient services: A.-General surgery, Dr. Warren Cole; B.-General Surgery, Dr. William Grove; and

C.-Thoracic and Cardiovascular, multiple attending staff. Each service had a senior resident and an assistant resident and I was the extra man. There was a little discomfort because every operation I did was one less operation for my fellow junior assistant resident. Although everyone wished to do as many operations as possible, I was tolerated and not made to feel redundant. Each service was quite busy, operating a full schedule and manning the outpatient clinics.

I enjoyed the technical aspects of the surgery, but did not like abdominal work; there always seemed to be an excess of intestines that one had to pack out of the way. The meticulous anatomical dissection in head and neck surgery, breast, thyroid, and thoracic surgery appealed to me. I operated often with Drs. Danley Slaughter and Harry Southwick, the surgical oncologists. Dr. Slaughter operated rapidly, applying multiple hemostats and never stopping until the specimen was removed. At that point, he would tell me to "dry it up and close" and left the OR. Dr. Southwick was a master technical cancer surgeon, using a scalpel to cut tissue away from the major vein in the arm when doing a radical mastectomy for breast cancer. The less talented did this with scissors, more slowly and with less precision. Although I found the technical challenge of head and neck cancer surgery of great interest, the post-operative morbidity and patient suffering seemed dreadful, and this did not seem an appropriate career.

I rotated on C. Service thoracic and vascular relatively early and scrubbed on virtually all of the heart operations. My chief resident did not wish to scrub because of the poor results achieved and patient complications. At that stage in the development of cardiac surgery, most of the operations were for congenital heart disease, using cardio-pulmonary bypass still in a developmental phase. Substantial progress had been made during my last year at the University of Minnesota, where their work with the heart-lung pump had been successful.

Our patients with small atrial septal defects repaired rapidly with a short pump run did well. The more complex ventricular septal defect and tetralogy patients requiring a longer bypass period did not awaken in the recovery room because of multiple small emboli in the brain related to the prolonged pump run. Dr. Ormand Julian, our cardiac surgeon, persisted realizing that the field was in development and required continued meticulous work. I lacked the background to have his perspective. The development of cardiac surgery for atherosclerotic disease was undeveloped and we were not doing coronary artery bypass.

I assisted Dr. Hushang Javid on what I believe was the first carotid endarterectomy performed in Chicago in 1957. C. Miller Fisher at the Massachusetts General Hospital did pathology studies demonstrating the importance of disease at the carotid bifurcation in the neck in stroke. This was clearly an important area for neurosurgery to explore. I later asked Dr. Oldberg to start a carotid surgery program, but he wanted Dr. Julian's cardio-vascular service to assume this function in the College of Medicine. This was a strategic mistake in the development of Neurosurgery in Chicago because we were not involved in much of the early stroke work. Fortunately, Dr. Francis Murphy in Memphis and Dr. Thor Sundt at the Mayo Clinic continued to make contributions in the treatment of carotid artery disease in the neck and, at the national level, kept neurosurgery involved in cerebrovascular disease.

Children having unsuccessful cardiac surgery were emotionally devastating. We had a 13-year-old boy on service that was building a balsa wood and paper model airplane. On evening rounds before surgery, the balsa wood frame was finished. Surgery was complex and long, and he did not survive. On late evening rounds that night, the plane was still at the bedside in his room. A crushing remembrance for the entire staff. That era in cardiac surgery was very difficult.

Gladys and I saw one another as time permitted. She was

working and attending DePaul University; both of us were extremely busy. We decided to marry in November when an apartment became available in the University Staff Apartment building. Gladys made the arrangements with the minister at the Chicago Temple, the Methodist Church on top of a downtown office building. We were married in the "Chapel in the Sky" an intimate small room containing 16 stained glass windows and seating 30 that had been created in 1952, only five years before. Dr. Cole did not entirely approve, feeling that the surgical residency was a full-time task not allowing time for marriage. The wedding was to occur at 11 a.m. Saturday and Dr. Cole requested that I meet with him in his office at 8 a.m. that day to review a paper I was to present to the Chicago Surgical Society the following week. We were finished by 9:30, I met Gladys at the church on time for our wedding, and we were both back to work at 6 a.m. Monday morning.

My career decision process was progressing; the poor results and seemingly long developmental period in heart surgery were discouraging. I did not like abdominal surgery, the main stay of general surgery, and excluded that career. Although I enjoyed the technical aspects of head and neck surgery, this was largely cancer surgery. The postoperative status of those that had radical neck dissections with excision of part of the jaw or tongue was disappointing. I lacked the necessary enthusiasm for surgery and the surgical subspecialties.

Although brain surgery was at a point requiring a great deal of technical improvement, the wonder of brain function overwhelmed all of my rational reasons against entering the field. I talked with Dr. Eric Oldberg, Professor and Head of the Neurosurgery Department about training in neurosurgery, and began to consider moving to the Illinois Neuropsychiatric Institute for the next stage of my career. Even though neurosurgery was "full", I took the chance that there would be a place to work after finishing.

Should I stay in Chicago for training or go further afield?

Where to Train? Exploring

My decision was made, I wanted to be a neurosurgeon and the next question was where to train? In 1956 there were relatively few good places to train in the United States, and most arrangements were made by private agreement with a mentor. In recent years, a formal matching program has resulted in a very transparent, democratic, and relatively efficient process for matching residents to the 100 programs available, but I confronted a much more opaque informal limited process.

Since my interest in neurosurgery had evolved after reading Dr. Wilder Penfield's work in epilepsy at the Montreal Neurological Institute, that was the first place to explore. At that time, the MNI gave one six months to become proficient in French, one of the immediate challenges to training in Montreal. I flew to Montreal and waited through the day to visit with Dr. Theodore Rasmussen, the service chief. I met Dr. Jasper, the electoencephalographer during the day, visited in neuropathology, neuroradiology, and neuro-chemistry and was impressed by the support system for doing neurological research. Dr. Rasmussen and I had tea in his office that evening, and he cautioned me that the fellows at the MNI were not the primary surgeon on most cases, except for indigent patients with a malignant tumor who were funded by the Province of Quebec. At that point, I very much wanted "hands on" surgical experience and that seemed distant at Montreal. Further exploration was necessary.

I flew to New York late that night, and the following day, went to 168th Street to visit the Neurological Institute of New York, a part of the Columbia Presbyterian Medical Center. Things were more informal in that era. Dr. J. Lawrence Pool, the neurosurgery chief, not only agreed to see me, he arranged interviews with three neurosurgeons and three neurologists over two days. After two days, he told me I could come next year but would have to spend a year on the neurology service with Dr. Houston Merritt, at that time one of the most famous neurologists in the world. Dr. Pool arranged an interview with Dr. Merritt across a library table in the NINY library on the 14th floor. Dr. Merritt was cordial, down to earth and kind. He arranged for me to meet with Dr. Sidney Carter, who at the time was developing pediatric neurology as a specialty in the United States. NINY was an exciting opportunity, but I left concerned about my ability to live in New York and wondering if I could manage a year in medical neurology—I wanted to continue operating!

The other center I considered was the University of Michigan led by Dr. Eddie Kahn, one of the leading Midwestern centers. I visited there and spent almost a day with Dr. Kahn. The most memorable event of the trip was a new instrument which he called "the pneumatic skull plow" (an early version of a pneumatic skull perforator). Previously, the burr holes to open the skull were placed with a brace and bit, which required a great deal of work. This machine used compressed air and was very fast and required little effort. However, with the first drill hole, the drill failed to stop and perforated the dura mater (the outer covering of the brain) and the right frontal lobe of the brain. Fortunately, brain damage was avoided because the perforation occurred in the tumor that was to be removed.

Dr. Kahn felt that I should have two more years of general surgery in preparation for neurosurgical training. Four years of preliminary training seemed inappropriate, making Michigan a poor fit for my career.

I meanwhile was busy as a general surgery senior intern at the Illinois Research and Educational Hospital. Any thoughts of cardiac surgery were rapidly leaving as I observed the morbidity and mortality of cardiac surgery at that stage of development. Dr.

Oldberg called and asked if I wanted a place at the University of Illinois. I could start neurosurgery immediately after the general surgery year, and Dr. Oldberg seemed disinclined to wait for my decision. I was anxious to immediately start operative neurosurgery; I told him the next day that I would stay in Chicago. The decision was made!

Chapter 3

Beginning a Life in Neuroscience 1957-1961

To learn one must be humble.
But life is the great teacher
—James Joyce, *Ulysses*

Neurosurgical Residency Begins

The length of the neurosurgical residency in 1957 was either 3 or 4 years after one or two years in general surgery. The American Board of Neurological Surgery required 30 months of clinical neurological surgery. At the University of Illinois, most residents completed three years after their general surgical training, comprising 30 months of clinical neurosurgery and six months of neuropathology. Neurosurgery residents provided all of the inpatient neurology care and neuroradiology. The University utilized the Neuropsychiatric Institute (NPI) of the Illinois Research and Educational Hospital (R&E), the neurosurgery service at Saint Luke's Hospital, The Presbyterian Hospital, and the Hines VA Hospital for their teaching program. The University of Illinois neurosurgery residents experienced various rotations in those hospitals.

The Neuropsychiatric Institute of the University of Illinois opened in 1941 on South Wood Street in the West side of Chicago. A large art deco building with twin towers, the north tower utilized for neurology and neurosurgery, and the south tower served psychiatry. The towers were connected at the first floor by clinics rather like the corpus callosum in the brain. The basement housed a large neurophysiology laboratory. Ralph Gerard, a neurophysiologist from the University of Chicago led the laboratory, replacing Warren McCulloch after he moved to MIT. As I entered the NPI, Drs. Oldberg, Sugar, and Percival Bailey led the clinical staff, and Dr. Leo Abood and Alex Geiger were in the laboratory. Dr. Fred and Erna Gibbs were doing pioneering work in EEG. Gerhardt von Bonin, the neuroanatomist, was working on the structure and function of the cerebral cortex. Dr. Roland MacKay and Ben Lichtenstein were the attending neurologists, and Dr. Francis Gerty led the Psychiatry Department. The structure and organization of the NPI reinforced my thinking about integrated neuroscience first generated by Penfield's work.

July 1, 1957, I began neurosurgical training as the sole neurosurgical resident at the Saint Luke's Hospital on South Michigan Avenue in Chicago, Dr. Oldberg's private service. I was responsible for the neurosurgery service at Saint Luke's 24 hours a day seven days a week and had a bedroom adjacent to the patient floor. Dr. Oldberg came daily to make rounds and to operate; occasionally the NPI chief resident accompanied him. I reported the status of the patients to Dr. Oldberg each day and was independently responsible much of the time. I saw all of the new patients and discussed them with Dr. Oldberg, wrote a note, and addressed the problem with the referring private physician. Many first- year experiences are vivid after almost 60 years.

Dr. Oldberg told me to perform a pneumoencephalogram on a patient believed to have a brain tumor. This involved a spinal puncture for replacement of a small amount of spinal fluid with air while the patient sat upright. X-rays of the head were obtained, and if the head were properly positioned, the air passed into the ventricles and cisterns of the brain. The distortion of the ventricles revealed the location of the brain tumor. I had never seen the procedure performed, so I quickly read about it.

At the scheduled time, I went to radiology, did the spinal tap, injected 15 cc of air, and the patient promptly fell over unconscious. She remained so for the longest 5 minutes I have experienced. She then awakened, inquired as to what had happened, and we took the x-rays which fortunately revealed the ventricles filled with enough air to make a diagnosis. I was now a neuroradiologist with "air study" experience. In the current era, a resident performs all procedures with supervision before functioning independently.

I had been at the hospital 90 days, and on Labor Day, Dr. Oldberg told me that I could take the afternoon off. Later that day, he sent a patient from Michigan that had a diving accident with a cervical spine fracture dislocation. He instructed me "put him in tongs". At that time, most cervical spine fractures were treated by placing tongs in the skull, attaching weights, and the resulting traction aligned the spinal dislocation. This was my first experience with Crutchfield tongs. Again, a quick read was necessary, and I placed the tongs using the drill supplied by the experienced nurse, and all went well.

Malignant brain tumors were usually diagnosed with an air study that made the brain swelling worse, and agents to control brain swelling or cerebral edema were unavailable. As a result after a biopsy of a glioblastoma multiforme (the common malignant brain tumor of adult life), the patient often became steadily worse and died in the early post-operative course. Since we were attempting to learn much more about this disease, an autopsy was performed on virtually every patient who expired on our service. I was responsible for the brain portion of the examination. The pathologists in the hospital never missed an opportunity to point out my frequent participation.

There was a single neurology resident at the hospital, Dr. Hernando Torres from Bogota, Columbia. We discussed neurology in the evening to while away the time. The two of us were essentially responsible for neurosurgery and neurology in the hospital for the year. Hernando subsequently trained in neurosurgery at the University of Chicago with Dr. Joe Evans and Dr. Sean Mullen. He was the first physician from another country to become a long time friend and colleague. Hernando gave me my first Basque beret that I wore for over 40 years until I was fortunate to find a replacement in Quebec City.

Residency training at that time was very different from today's program, and there was much more program variation. Program requirements were not well defined, and the accreditation process was not rigorous. I was immediately totally responsible for the well-being of the patients and did not have a cadre of fellow residents, and none more senior. New problems were often my first experience, and I did not know entirely what to expect. I visited patients frequently, through the night, to assure myself that all was well when in unfamiliar territory. Thankfully, modern residency programs provide progressive supervised responsibility.

The total resident and faculty cadre was appreciably smaller than today's departments. Essentially all of the attending functions were performed by Dr. Oldberg and Dr. Oscar Sugar, with an occasional visiting physician. Physician Assistants and Advanced Practice Nurses were in the distant future. The 52-bed service at the NPI was managed by three residents and an intern. The attending faculty made rounds once or twice a week, and the residents cared for the patients the remainder of the time. Most university neurosurgery departments had a small faculty, and the resident group was also small. In Minneapolis, Dr. Peyton and Dr. French were the core staff for the University of Minnesota service. Neurosurgery departments with ten to twenty neurosurgeons and 14 to 21 residents are now commonplace.

NPI, "The Chief Resident"

July 1, 1958, after trial by fire for a year, I entered my second year at the Neuropsychiatric Institute assisted by a junior resident, and an intern. Life was much better with a room on the 8th floor, for my convenience and call every third night. My junior resident Phil Lippe had been in the military, yet did not entirely understand that I outranked him. Phil listed tasks on his clip board for me to perform initially, and this was soon clarified.

Dr. Oldberg called me to his office the day before Christmas. I would become "Chief" on January 1, 1960, after I had been a resident 18 months. Protesting that I was not ready, Dr. Oldberg responded "you are ready". Later that day, two residents preceding me in the program were told that they were not ready to be chief resident and were assigned to other hospitals. Again, a great deal of reading and preparation was required. I remained "Chief", with the exception of six months in the pathology laboratory with Dr. Bailey, for the remainder of my residency.

The nature of the workload was very different than neurosurgical practice today. The NPI served as a neurological hospital for the medically indigent of Illinois, and occasionally for non-indigent patients with an inordinately complex problem such as conjoined twins. The bulk of the work involved a brain tumor operation, daily, interspersed with temporal lobe resections for epilepsy, and stereotactic operations for Parkinson's disease. Little spinal surgery was performed; virtually all of these patients were cared for in the private sector. The University of Illinois Research and Educational Hospital lacked an active emergency room thus Cook County Hospital assumed responsibility for trauma. Carotid endarterectomy was assigned to the cardiovascular service and spine fusions to orthopedic surgery.

Finishing residency I was confident performing frontal craniotomy for a pituitary tumor. This was an uncommon problem in private neurosurgical practice. The operation was done extradural to the sphenoid wing as Harvey Cushing had performed that operation after he ceased doing the nasal transsphenoidal operation. Although Gerard Guiot in Paris was operating upon pituitary tumors via a nasal transsphenoidal route, neurosurgeons in the United States still utilized a craniotomy.

Temporal lobe epilepsy resections with depth electrode recording under local anesthesia were performed with methods similar to the Montreal procedure. Dr. Percival Bailey developed the program and Dr. Fred Gibbs was our electoencephalographer. The operations took much of the day, and Dr. Gibbs came to the operating room while we were doing the recording from the brain surface and depth electrodes. The long operations under local anesthesia exhausted the patient and the surgeon.

Although lumbar disc operations were quite rare, we operated on a number of intramedullary (tumor within the spinal cord) spinal tumors, probably because the physicians in the private sector were somewhat reluctant to do them. Oligodendrogliomas with a discrete margin could be removed quite well by a skilled surgeon. Astrocytomas blended into the normal spinal cord and could not be entirely removed. As usual, Dr. Oldberg entered the room after I exposed the spinal cord. He raised his hand, the nurse placed the fine scalpel, and he incised the spinal cord. With very fine forceps, he dissected the tumor away from the surrounding spinal cord in twenty minutes, dropped the specimen in the pan, instructing, "close Pat, I will be in the office". He never assisted, operated rapidly without loupe magnification with little morbidity, and seemed to welcome the challenge of this operation. A virtuoso performance in the era antedating the surgical microscope.

Stereotactic surgery for Parkinson's disease was performed utilizing local anesthesia. The globus pallidus and thalamic procedures began with a small air study to identify the third ventricle and anterior and posterior commissure for anatomical targeting of the lesion. Polaroid film saved time lost in waiting for X-ray images. The optimum patients were young people with unilateral tremor. Excellent results were achieved in that small group of patients with a profound unilateral rest tremor. These operations with the patient awake were at times dramatic. When the probe struck the target, the tremor would cease before the lesion was made. I did one or two stereotactic operations each week when Dr. Gustafson, the attending surgeon, was available Levo Dopa was not yet available as a medical therapy, and we were the only center in Chicago doing this procedure.

The neurosurgical staff did all of the neuro-radiology; the usual arrangement at that time in the United States. Sweden and the United Kingdom had well-developed neuro-radiology with trained radiology subspecialists. This transition was just beginning in the United States, with Dr. Juan Taveras doing pioneering neuroradiology in New York. In Chicago in the '50s, neuroradiology was done primarily by neurosurgeons who were reluctant to relinquish their role. I performed carotid and vertebral angiography with a percutaneous needle, obtaining three films with each injection because we had not acquired Swedish film changers. We simply numbed the skin, inserted an 18 gauge needle in the carotid or vertebral artery, and injected the contrast material, calling to the technician "shoot" to capture the image at the optimum time.

All myelography (spinal canal contrast imaging) was achieved without image intensification to enhance the image. A spinal tap was done in the lumbar region and we introduced a lipid (oil) based contrast agent that had to be removed after the films were obtained. The contrast agent allowed imaging of the contents of the spinal canal. Removal of the contrast agent invariably caused pain shooting into the leg or perineum if a nerve root was aspirated. Aspiration of the contrast agent required an 18 gauge spinal needle, almost invariably leading to intense post-spinal puncture headaches, lasting several days. Wearing red goggles, for several hours before the procedure, enhanced our visual function. Even with this technique, the fluoroscopic image was poor. Multiple spot film images were obtained during the fluoroscopic study. We were unsure about the result until these films were developed and complete review accomplished. Myelography was an unpleasant experience that few patients were willing to repeat.

Air studies were done either with a lumbar puncture (pneumoencephalogram) or by direct bilateral ventricular puncture (ventriculogram) through a burr hole in the skull. These studies were first done at the Johns Hopkins Hospital by Dr. Walter Dandy, the chief of neurosurgery. X-ray films revealed air entering the various fluid-filled spaces in the brain. The distortions indirectly indicated the location of the tumor. We preformed ventriculograms in the operating room with the patient awake. The posterior scalp was numbed with Novocain on each side, and a small opening made in the skull with a drill. We then put a needle into the brain about 2.5-3 inches until striking the ventricle, indicated by CSF coming out of the needle. A tumor frequently displaced the ventricle from its usual position making it difficult to strike the ventricle. These procedures were done early in the morning with the operation immediately after the ventriculogram study. The air study changed the intracranial dynamics, with significant worsening of the patient's condition as brain swelling increased, in the hours after the study.

Intensive care or intermediate care units did not exist. The patients recovered in the operating room, then were transferred to a room on the floor near the nursing desk. Anesthesiologists rotated from the general hospital, and the need for specialized expertise in neurological anesthesia was not recognized.

Neurological surgery residents were appointed both in neurology and neurological surgery and were responsible for all neurological consultations. A neurology resident was rarely appointed and the faculty neurologists, Dr. Roland McKay, Dr. Jay Garvin, Dr. Ben Lichtenstein, and Dr. Louis Boshes all functioned largely in the outpatient clinics. The inpatient service was the domain of the neurosurgeons. The neurosurgery residents did all of the neuro-ophthalmology including tangent screen visual field examinations. This was essentially how Dr. Harvey Cushing managed the Brigham Hospital service and Dr. Oldberg emulated his custom. He felt that a neurosurgeon must be a competent neurologist, neuro-ophthalmologist, and neuroradiologist as well as a neurosurgeon.

I was conducting a clinical research trial with a copper chelating agent for Wilson's disease. Wilson's disease is a metabolic disease involving copper metabolism causing liver disease and brain basal ganglia malfunction with tremor. Although some patients had significant liver disease, because of the referral patterns to a neurological center, most of my patients had tremor and other extrapyramidal signs. Participation in this clinical trial provided an opportunity to acquire expertise in a rare disease.

Neurology and neurosurgery care was totally integrated, and there were few neurology faculty. We consulted on inpatients with myasthenia, multiple sclerosis, muscular dystrophy, and peripheral neuropathy. We rarely were asked to see a stroke patient, considered patients of the medicine service.

Children with myelodysplasia (spina bifida), hydrocephalous, and chronic subdural hematoma filled the twelve-bed pediatric unit. Chronic subdual hematoma, liquid blood clots over the surface of the brain, was a common problem that became less frequent with improved obstetrical management. Initially, we were placing the hydrocephalous shunt in the ureter. Late in my residency, I placed the first Pudenz ventriculo-jugular shunt in Chicago in 1959. Later the shunt was placed in the right atrium of the heart as the result of our experience with thrombosis in the jugular vein.

Vascular neurosurgery was in its infancy and Dr. Oscar Sugar was developing a new program at the NPI. Patients with subarachnoid hemorrhage were kept in a quiet room for 1-2 weeks then had carotid angiography. If carotid angiography was negative, only then did vertebral angiography follow. Posterior communicating and ophthalmic aneurysms were treated with carotid occlusion with a Salibi clamp on the common carotid in the neck, a modification of the Selverstone clamp, with a significant number of patients developing paralysis on the opposite side of the body. A few anterior communicating and middle cerebral aneurysms were treated with either silver Olivecrona clips or ligatures placed on the neck of the aneurysm. Clips that were readily removed were not available, the initial clip placement was usually the final clip placement. These operations were done with loupe magnification and headlight. The results were often poor because of injury to unseen tiny perforating vessels.

Because Dr. Oldberg wished Dr. Ormand Julian of the cardio-vascular surgery to develop carotid surgery, I worked in the animal lab developing skills in cervical carotid surgery. I felt this would become an important part of neurosurgery. The care of stoke patients was not attracting the interest of neuroscience physicians in the '50s.

Relatively few peripheral nerve problems came to the service. Lord Brain in England described the carpal tunnel syndrome in 1947, and we were beginning to see patients with profound atrophy of muscle in the thumb and weakness of opposition of the thumb and little finger caused by median nerve compression at the carpal tunnel in the wrist. A few carpal tunnel operations were done by the neurosurgery service, but most were referred to the hand service in general surgery.

Ward rounds with Dr. Oldberg and/or Dr. Sugar were teaching and work rounds. Residents wore spotless lab coats, neckties and shined shoes. Presentations were brief, organized with all perti-nent positives and negatives. Bedside presentations began with patient's dominant hand and occupation, and the chronology of the illness was precise. Appropriate laboratory and imaging results were presented, and any unnecessary tests had to be justi-fied to the attending staff. Critical neurological findings were assessed, and management decisions completed on 52 patients in several hours.

I had finished 2 years of preliminary clinical work, largely general and specialty surgery, 2.5 years of neurosurgery, and six months of neuropathology. I was a relatively experienced brain tumor surgeon but had only a modicum of spine surgery expe-rience. Today, the neurosurgical residency lasts seven years, and the spectrum of neurosurgery is immensely greater. Academic neurosurgery departments in the '50s declined funds offered by the NIH to expand programs and research, unlike neurology departments who sought NIH support. The result was a paucity of research in neurosurgery departments, few full-time faculty, and in most programs, little research training. In retrospect, the decision of academic neurosurgery to not embrace NIH programs was unwise and failed to appreciate the potential for dramatic improvement. A conservative approach delayed growth of faculty and resident programs in neurosurgery.

The NPI program provided good clinical preparation, but neither prepared or encouraged me to pursue an academic career. In many respects, the residency shared the strengths and deficiencies of the University Of Illinois College of Medicine; a pragmatic preparation for medicine as it was, rather than for what was to come. Early in my subsequent academic career, I understood that faculty were responsible for making students aware of diverse career opportunities. Significant mentoring to support the optimum career for their trainees must be integrated. Much later, I would have an opportunity to demonstrate my own inadequacy in that role.

Dr. Oldberg failed to develop research talent and academic leadership but brought a unique human value to the program. His residents became thoughtful, competent compassionate clinicians because he would tolerate nothing less. He insisted on consistent accuracy in diagnosis and treatment avoiding inappropriate and unnecessary testing. Precise comprehensive analysis with absolute intellectual honesty was his expectation. Patients and family were treated with the utmost respect and kindness. The neurosurgery residents and staff were the most obviously professional staff in the R and E Hospital, with necktie, spotless white coat, and polished shoes and an ophthalmoscope and reflex hammer in their coat pocket.

Dr. Oldberg had wide-ranging interests (President of the

59

Chicago Symphony, The Chicago Board of Health, etc.) and he expected that from his trainees. He once told me, he dreaded the national neurosurgery meetings, because they were filled with neurosurgeons with remarkably circumscribed interests. Dr. Oldberg liked to talk with multi-dimensional people and was a member of The Cliff Dwellers Club in Chicago. He often took the Chief resident and his wife to the Club for dinner above Symphony Hall. The members of The Cliff Dwellers were musicians, artists, and authors. The painting were the work of the members, and the books were written by the members. As president of the Chicago Symphony, his box was in the midline at Symphony Hall, above the conductor. When away from the city, he gave the Chief resident the box. I would read Claudia Cassidy's critique of the symphony performance in the Chicago Tribune, because an unfavorable review predicted a bad day with the "Chief". Saturday surgery was finished by 1:00 p.m. because he played bridge at the Chicago Club, shortly thereafter. He looked forward to the intellectual challenge. Dr. Oldberg told me I had two deficiencies; bridge and baseball. He loved going to Wrigley Field summer afternoons. He was physician and friend to Mayor Richard Daley. Dr. Oldberg was very much a citizen of Chicago.

Spina Bifida, Lifelong Care Begins

Kyle Crown was admitted to the NPI second floor pediatric unit, transferred from downstate Illinois, where he was born several days earlier. Kyle was the first child of young parents who lived in Elmwood, Illinois, a small town west of Peoria. At birth, a small midline sac was noted on his back just below the waist. An opening in the sac drained a small amount of clear CSF (cerebrospinal fluid). The State of Illinois Division of Services for Crippled Children (DSCC) arranged transfer to the Illinois NPI. Examination on admission revealed a slightly enlarged head and the sac in the midline on his back about 1.5 inches in size. The left lower leg did not move well, and urine drained when he cried, indicating impaired bladder control.

The diagnosis was lumbosacral myelomeningocele with hydrocephalous, a congenital failure of closure of the lower end of the spinal canal, often associated with Arnold-Chiari malformation (a congenital defect involving the brain stem causing hydrocephalous). The sac broke during delivery, was draining, and presented the threat of infection of the cerebrospinal fluid, meningitis with death or serious disability. I operated to close the defect that night. Surgery went well, and his ability to move his legs was unchanged the following morning. His fontanel or soft spot became tight and the wound was puffy, indicating that the hydrocephalous must be treated.

I returned Kyle to surgery the following day placing one of the new Pudenz ventriculoatrial shunts to control the hydrocephalous. This tubing allowed the excess fluid in the ventricles of the brain to pass into the blood stream in the heart. The shunt procedure immediately controlled the problem, and Kyle was able to return home in ten days. His incisions were healed but he continued to have a problem with bladder control. Moderate weakness remained in the left foot and a little weakness was present in the right foot. This remained a difficult problem for Kyle's mother and father, but his mother was determined to provide everything Kyle needed. He was to be seen in follow-up by a pediatrician in Peoria, and in our clinic in six months.

Within six months I had arrived in Peoria, and, somehow, his determined mother made the connection to my practice. Soon Kyle was in my office, and a relationship began that endured for 35 years. Walking developed more slowly than with other children because bracing was needed, and he required supervision by a urologist. On a number of occasions, his hydrocephalous shunt became plugged and required emergency revision, because of a severe headache followed by drowsiness. With one of the revisions, the distal shunt was removed from the heart and placed in the abdomen, a location associated with fewer complications. Ultimately Kyle walked with two Canadian crutches, was employed, and married.

Over the subsequent years in Peoria, I was called to the newborn nursery multiple times to confront a similar problem. As prenatal testing developed, the presence of a myelomeningocele was no longer a surprise at delivery but always, was a very complex heart breaking challenge to young parents. Care of these children steadily improved, as we developed a multidisciplinary team involving neurosurgeons, neurologists, orthopedic surgeons, urologists, and pediatricians, all with an interest in these children. I became aware of the stress on the patient and parents caused by frequent visits to multiple doctors and established a clinic allowing children to see the specialists in one visit. Working with the DSCC, we established a myelodysplasia clinic with the Children's Hospital. Mrs. Mildred Miller, an experienced, dedicated pediatric nurse, accepted the leadership of the clinic and we provided care for these children in a large area of Downstate Illinois.

In most cases, there was no identified cause for the birth defect, with only an occasional specific causative factor such as several medications taken by the mother during pregnancy. We were seeing about one new patient per month until 1991-2 when a significant breakthrough occurred. It was reported early in the *Lancet* from the United Kingdom, (1) and later in the *New England Journal of Medicine* (2) that taking folic acid prevented neural tube defects, reducing the incidence by one half. There was an immediate public health effort to assure that women were taking folate before conception. There has been a significant reduction in incidence with this measure. This improvement is another dramatic example of the value of clinical research in population health. A relatively simple and inexpensive action prevents much human suffering.

The most recent development is the advent of fetal surgery for neural tube defects. Children with this diagnosis on ultrasound are now considered for surgery during the pregnancy. The fetus is taken out of the uterus briefly, the neural tube defect closed, and the fetus returned to the uterus. It is claimed that the extent of paralysis is decreased and fewer children require hydrocephalous shunting. This procedure is done in six centers in the United States, and data regarding outcome continues to be collected. This procedure requires further critical study. (3)

Finishing: What to Do Now?

On graduation from medical school in 1956, the government offered the Berry Plan providing deferment from the military draft for specialty training. The plan required specialty practice in the military for a minimum of two years at residency completion. The Berry Plan was intended to solve a perceived problem of an inadequate supply of medical specialists for the armed forces. Eight army neurosurgery centers required surgical staff. The Army office in Chicago informed me there was no assigned position in the spring of 1961 as I finished training. Only the Army Medical Department staff in Washington could provide the plan for my military future.

I arrived in Washington; found the needed department, (interestingly, in the Navy building) and walked into a large room filled with majors and colonels, all sitting at desks piled with papers. Two neurosurgeons had already decided to stay in the regular Army meeting the Army's need for the next several years. An opportunity to join a laboratory performing surgery on monkeys in the Army Chemical Warfare Program was offered but not mandated. Clinical medicine was my interest; the Army told me I must find a position in an Army Reserve unit. A unit in Saint Louis agreed to take a man with my background on the condition that I not complicate their budget by attending meetings. The reserve career ended in 1968 when I received a letter from the Army informing me that I had not achieved promotion by active participation in the reserve unit. I was discharged from the US Army Reserve. At that time, I had three small children, an all-consuming practice, and I was draft eligible. The first letter was soon followed by another informing me I was too old for military duty.

About 600 neurosurgeons were practicing in the United States and the large metropolitan areas were deemed to be "full". Opportunities in spine surgery were in the future, and cerebrovascular surgery was in its infancy. There were three neurosurgeons in downstate Illinois; Dr. Floyd Barringer in Springfield, Dr. Lawrence Holden in Peoria, and Dr. John Van Landingham in Rockford serving five million people. Although the Downstate was clearly "full of neurosurgeons", returning home seemed attractive. Brain surgery was my all-consuming interest and Dr. Holden enjoyed spinal surgery. A natural fit! My career as a "country neurosurgeon "was to begin.

Chapter 4

A Neurological Center
1961-1970

I wanted real adventures to happen to myself. But real adventures, I reflected, do not happen to people who remain at home: they must be sought abroad.

—James Joyce, *Dubliners*

July 23, 1961:
Beginning Neurosurgical Practice

Having decided to develop a neurosurgical practice in my hometown, Gladys and I rented a small apartment five minutes from the hospital. In that era, the surgeons provided the surgical instruments. Our savings were expended by purchasing a $5000 set of neurosurgical instruments. The residual savings bought a used stove and refrigerator for the apartment. I arranged a sublet of an examining room and hired a part-time secretary, Mary Cody, from Dr. Paul Palmer, an industrial physician in Peoria. The initial practice overhead was $30 per month in the Jefferson Building downtown. Gladys typed the letters to referring physicians at night on our new IBM Selectric typewriter, avoiding a secretarial salary. We were up and running!

The first day three new patients appeared, all referred by Dr. Palmer. Each patient had injured their lumbar spine at work and did not wish an early return to employment. This was an auspicious start for the brain surgery program, I envisioned. Within weeks, I had operated upon several patients for a lumbar herniated disc, seemingly the major and perhaps only neurosurgical problem in Central Illinois.

Dr. Larry Holden was Peoria's first neurosurgeon, having moved from the Illinois NPI in Chicago in 1949. I met him before coming to Peoria, and he welcomed my arrival and was encouraging. Larry was not interested in a partnership. He enjoyed his practice as it was, and was confident that I would be busy on arrival. Larry grew up on a dairy farm in upper New York State, near Syracuse, and came to the University of Illinois in Urbana to become an engineer. One summer, after talking to a pre-med student, he changed his mind and decided that medicine might be more fun. He was faithful to his roots and was the only neurosurgeon who read the *Journal of Neurosurgery* and *Hoard's Dairyman*, the professional journal equivalent of the dairy industry.

Although innovative and creative with an exceptionally curious intellect, he never was certified in neurosurgery because he did not see the point of the examination or the certification process, implemented in August 1940. There were a number of practicing neurosurgeons that failed to take the board examination. It did not seem to have limited Dr. Holden's career.

Larry's primary interest was spinal disorders, and mine was intracranial problems, so we complemented one another. He enjoyed his eccentricities immensely. He played bridge and often disappeared to the back of the Rex Radiator Shop, a den for bridge and poker, where few could find him. Larry purchased a 1949 two passenger, all-aluminum Luscombe airplane, shortly after coming to Peoria. He loved to fly into farm fields and land in unconventional locations. A master of "slipping" the plane into rural pastures, he always avoided the cows. The Luscombe was utilized to see rural consultations. The referring physician picked him up at the local airport or a farm field. Later he acquired a twin- engine Piper Comanche, nicknamed "the widow maker" because of its performance characteristics. This was a much faster plane that extended the range of his wanderings. He continued always to ask if we wanted to fly over or under large river bridges, while touring Illinois.

One morning, Dr. Charles Branch, the Chief Medical Officer at Saint Francis Hospital, called to tell me Dr. Holden was riding his motorcycle down the 800 B neurosurgery ward hall with Mrs. Anna May Lightbody, the head nurse, riding pillion. Charlie wanted my plan for dealing with the problem. I had none. Although at times, Larry's eccentricities were maddening, he was always supportive, always willing to talk over or assist on a difficult problem and contributed to my relative sanity in the 1961 — 1968 period of solo neurosurgical practice. Larry was compassionate and scrupulously honest with others and himself. Without his presence, the intellectual isolation in that seven-year period would have been difficult to endure. Larry died early of heart disease at sixty-eight. I miss his presence, encouragement, and unpredictable behavior.

The first brain tumor patient was referred for a back problem but proved to have a parasagittal meningioma, and the brain program began! After a year sharing Dr. Palmer's office in the Jefferson building, I was ready to have my own office. A 900 square foot office was designed on the third floor of the downtown Jefferson Building. We used pocket doors to decrease the square footage required in the examining rooms, creating a very efficient space. This office served well from 1962 until October 1966, when on the day of my youngest son John's birth, the office was moved to a new building adjacent to Saint Francis Hospital at 416 Saint Mark Court.

Fortunately, there was a serious shortage of neurological care in the entire downstate area, and the practice became very busy. Referring physicians had little understanding of the specific role of neurologists and neurosurgeons. I saw patients with multiple sclerosis, Parkinson's disease, headache, seizures, and children with a learning disability. After a year, a senior pediatrician, stopped me to ask if air studies were done in our hospital. I assured him that we had air in Peoria. There was a consistent tendency to send all significant problems to Barnes Hospital, Washington University in Saint Louis, or the Mayo Clinic, with occasional referrals to Chicago. I made a diagnosis of craniopharyngioma in a young woman, examined by her primary physician, without a diagnosis for a number of months. I called him with my diagnosis and plan; he immediately informed the family they must go to the Mayo Clinic! Local commitment to specialty care was still in its infancy.

Initially, anesthesia was unavailable in the morning. Four anesthesiologists served the city, and the schedule was full of elective patients until 1-2 in the afternoon. I saw patients in the clinic each morning, and began surgery in the afternoon, and operated in the morning on Saturday and Sunday. The first several years, a referring physician often served as the assistant surgeon, and the scrub team lacked specialized knowledge of the instrumentation, impeding the progress of the surgery. Dr. Holden frequently assisted complex intracranial surgery.

The absence of a paging system required frequent calls to the answering service to determine if any emergencies were in progress. This arrangement added a bit of tension to the out of Peoria excursions. There was often 60-90 minutes when I was out of contact with the hospital operators. Picnics and other events were interrupted by repeated trips to public telephone booths. Physicians troubled today by being connected without interruption have not experienced this primitive lack of connectivity. Constantly connected seems a luxury after enduring years of seeking out public phone booths.

Developing a Neurological Center

Arriving in Peoria in July 1961, I was expected to work at all three hospitals; Saint Francis, Methodist, and Proctor Hospital. Saint Francis and Methodist were adjacent to one another downtown and served a similar role in the community; Proctor was a small new hospital in the north side. Dr. Holden was on the active staff at Methodist with Dr. Bruce Ehmke, the sole neurologist. Two types of staff appointment existed; active and courtesy. Active members participated in the full activity of the hospital with a vote on staff issues, courtesy members admitted patients but did not participate in the governance of the program and were nonvoting. I was born in the Methodist hospital, had attended the Methodist church in the country, and assumed that I would work at the Methodist Hospital on my return. Active staff appointment was by invitation and the expected invitation to join the active medical staff did not arrive. After a few months, I inquired about the lack of the desired invitation. The administration provided a prompt reply "Dr. Holden is on the active staff and one neurosurgeon is enough for a hospital". An interesting concept.

The Saint Francis Hospital was administered by Sister Canisa and associate administrator Ed McGrath. Although cautious, both were willing to commit to developing untried, early technology, if evidence suggested a reasonable chance of success. Their commitment to carefully considered proposals allowed utilization of new technology, early in development, and they did not have a neurosurgeon; an opportunity was apparent.

My patients were admitted to the orthopedic floor; the need for a neurological floor had not surfaced. Critical care units would be a future development. I used any available operating room, a specialized room was deemed unnecessary for neurosurgery. All units were staffed by nurses and technicians with general medical-surgical training. It was deemed pointless to develop facilities for a low volume service with little potential. It was apparent that a specialized unit would have to be created rather rapidly, if complex neurosurgery was to be accomplished safely. This task was achieved in the ensuing twenty years in a piecemeal fashion, much more slowly than I desired.

The first opportunity to develop a neurological center was the closure of the 8th floor 26-bed psychiatry unit. I asked Sister Canisa if she would consider conversion to a neuroscience unit. Creative use of unutilized space was appealing, and she approved without a business plan, further consultation, or feasibility studies. Shortly after that, the husband of a patient with a severe head injury provided funding for a specialized room next to the nursing desk for the most seriously ill patients, our first ICU bed. Poor elevator access and an inefficient architectural pattern resulted in an imperfect nursing unit, but the unit created an identified destination for neurological patients for the first time. Anna Mae Lightbody, RN, became the head nurse, and gradually developed a cadre of nurses knowledgeable in neurological care. Anna Mae selected staff that were dedicated and enjoyed caring for patients requiring complex care. She ruled with an iron hand in the style of an earlier era. Nursing staff liked the spirit and morale on 8B. The first step in developing a neurological center had been taken.

The medical staff lacked an organization supporting the care of neurological patients. The neurosurgeons were appointed in the surgery department, and Dr. Ehmke, the sole neurologist, served in the medicine department. When I first proposed a neuroscience department, the president of the medical staff opined that a department was unnecessary. There were only three neurological staff members, one active member, and little perceived potential or need for neuroscience development. Creation of a neuroscience department did require repeated visits to medical staff leadership over several years. A specialty neuroscience administrative structure was a critical step to achieve future growth and development.

Over thirty years, clinical growth created demand for additional facilities. A 26-bed 300B unit on the third floor followed. A large acute neurology floor, a neurological critical care unit, an adjacent intermediate unit, and an inpatient neurological rehabilitation unit all followed over several decades, culminating in a 100-bed Neurological Institute. The initial development was possible with the support of Sister Canisa and Mr. McGrath who were more adventuresome and visionary than the medical staff.

A Dedicated Operating Room

The first years an operating room was assigned as one became available. We operated late in the afternoon, after the more elective services had finished, working with a variety of nursing staff lacking neurosurgical experience. An OR early in the day, a team

71

of nurses familiar with brain surgery, and adequate lighting and space for the limited specialized equipment available at that time were all essential, urgently needed elements for an intracranial surgery program. Dr. Charles Branch, the Chief of Surgery, retired from clinical work several years after my arrival, releasing time in OR 1 for neurosurgical procedures. A dedicated surgical technician was assigned for the first time, providing consistency in operating room support.

OR 1 was a relatively small room, but adequate, and the room identification was the first acknowledgment that neurosurgery was a specialty, requiring special facilities. Lighting was dependent on the OR lights and a headlamp with a mirror and an incandescent bulb, providing inadequate light, while making my forehead uncomfortably warm. We acquired an early primitive fiber optic headlight, a striking improvement; a cool forehead with bright light was an incredible luxury. It is interesting to recall this long-ago concern with light. In that era, illuminating narrow, deep corridors in the brain was quite difficult. We used brain retractors with small light bulbs on the end that were immediately ineffective in the presence of any bleeding. The bleeding surrounded the light bulb, extinguishing all light at the most critical moments.

Magnification was added with a set of Keeler optical loupes I obtained from London. The next significant step was the first neurosurgical microscope in Illinois, described in the next chapter. Relatively soon, a craniotome (pneumatic skull perforator) became commercially available for $1000 and we were the first one in Illinois to acquire this apparatus. Unlike academic neurosurgical units, residents were not available to help with the work of opening the skull. This instrument provided much-appreciated relief from the physical stress involved in opening the skull for brain tumor operations. Before the craniotome, elevating the skull involved drilling multiple holes with a brace and bit, then connecting them with a Gigli saw, a wire saw with teeth. After an hour of carpentry, the actual brain operation could begin.

It was not possible to operate in the morning, because the limited anesthesiology time available was assigned on a first come, first served basis, and general surgery and tooth extractions were planned months in advance, securing all of the morning operative slots. The first several years virtually all major brain operations began in the afternoon or were done on Saturday when other services had finished their elective schedules. This did introduce a fatigue factor in long, complex operations. Nevertheless, the four anesthesiologists provided excellent anesthesia resulting in less anxiety about anesthesia mishaps than I experienced in Chicago.

Operating room 1 initiated a long process of developing excellent operating room facilities. More operating rooms were required as the neurosurgical staff increased. Next was the formation of a neurosurgical operating room team; skilled nurses committed to taking call, assuring an expert staff 24/7/365. The administration of Saint Francis Hospital committed to this potentially precedent-setting policy. Specialty teams were non-existent in Peoria, this was a major change requiring courage on the part of hospital leadership. Perhaps now, everyone would request a team creating an administrative nightmare.

The team was simply too small to distribute call assignment for nights and weekends. I proposed that the team serve the three hospitals in the community, substantially increasing the volume and size of the team. Saint Francis Hospital employed the team, and a contract with Methodist and Proctor paid an hourly rate, creating essentially an income-neutral state with benefit to all parties. This required unprecedented hospital cooperation. Neurosurgery had excellent operative support, the three hospitals had consistent OR coverage, and the cost structure provided value. This unusual cooperative state existed for many years until the thought of cooperating with competitors became intolerable, and the citywide program was disbanded. The model of a specialty team serving 2-5 hospitals is an effective concept for metropolitan areas with a population of 150-500,000. This strategy has not been widely adopted in the United States.

With the maturity of the neurosurgery residency program in 2016, 3 or 4 faculty surgeons and their residents operate daily. Neurosurgeons often utilize two rooms for optimum productivity. The surgeon is always present in the room during the essential portion of the operation. The operating room physical plant is the least expensive element in the OR equation, with staff and surgeon time utilization being the major cost structure determinants. Creation of an OR requires planning and negotiation because the number of OR's is limited by the Illinois certificate of need process. The neurosurgical service now often utilizes one room at Methodist and three at Saint Francis. We, like most services, struggle to achieve consistency in on-time starts and turn around between cases. Lost time increases OR costs and wastes surgeon time. It is distressing to know that Southwest Airline can turn around an airplane faster than we can turn over an OR. This indicates a lack of commitment to process evaluation and improvement by all elements involved. Deming's influence on manufacturing has not prevailed in health care.

Anesthesia

On my arrival, anesthesia was a relatively new medical specialty provided by four talented anesthesiologists serving the city. Dr. McQuiston, the senior member of the group, provided anesthesia for Dr. Pott's cardiac surgery program at Children's Memorial in Chicago, commuting virtually every week. Nurse anesthetists provided most of the anesthesia, but I attempted to have an anesthesiologist for my craniotomies.

Many neurosurgical procedures were performed with local anesthesia in US centers, and we often used these techniques.

Ventriculograms and burr holes for subdural hematoma were done with local anesthesia. Retrogasserian neurectomy for trigeminal neuralgia facial pain was also performed with local anesthesia. Testing the patient to ascertain sensory loss in the desired area of the face before closing the incision assured a satisfactory result. I performed brain tumor operations in critical brain areas with the patient awake for functional testing minimizing the risk of loss of brain function. This required gentle technique and patience. If a seizure occurred during the procedure, I irrigated the brain with iced saline and the seizure usually promptly stopped. Operations for temporal lobe epilepsy on the dominant language function hemisphere were often done with the patient awake. Speech and memory function could be tested before and during the brain tissue removal.

Local anesthesia was used for some spinal procedures as well. Dr. Holden, utilizing techniques learned from Dr. Semmes and Dr. Murphy in Memphis, did almost all of his lumbar and cervical disc operations with local anesthesia. I used general anesthesia for most disc operations, because I believed that intraoperative testing did not improve care. We frequently performed a proce-dure called cordotomy for severe pain in the spine and leg, most often caused by extensive cervical cancer in women. This required incision of the lateral spinothalamic pain pathway in the front of the upper thoracic spinal cord. The objective was to remove the ability to feel pain while preserving motion and position sense. The operation was performed under local anesthesia, with the patient resting prone, on pillows. The incision was in the midline, between the shoulder blades. After a tiny incision was made in the pain pathway in the spinal cord, the drapes were lifted, and I tested the patient's sensation with a safety pin. With the patient awake, I could be assured that the loss of pain sensation was adequate before finishing the operation. If the sensory loss was inadequate, I made a slightly larger incision while testing to ensure the motor pathways, immediately in back of the incision were not injured, and leg movement remained intact. Astounding progress in the care of carcinoma of the cervix and in pain management made cordotomy obsolete. A testament to remarkable medical progress in the care of cervical cancer.

Local anesthesia required changes in surgical technique and a culture change in the OR. The patient had to be well informed regarding the process, preparing him/her for each step of the surgery, avoiding surprises and actions that would enhance their anxiety. Unnecessary talk or noise frightening the patient was scrupulously avoided. The local anesthetic was injected slowly to decrease pain. Long procedures required repetition of the anesthetic injection. Incision and dissection were done with sharp cutting, avoiding tension and pulling that generated pain. I used a scalpel to take the muscles away from the spinous processes and lamina in the spine to avoid pain. The brain has no pain fibers, I only needed to prevent tension on blood vessels that caused pain. Local anesthetic was necessary around blood vessels in the dura covering the brain.

Although all of these changes in technique were necessary, and the patient found lying quietly for long periods difficult, there were critical practical advantages. The patients usually were free of nausea, could eat early after surgery, and moved about more rapidly. One could also test their brain and spinal cord function immediately, nothing was obscured by anesthesia and muscle relaxants.

Anesthesia improved rapidly with the training of many anesthesiologists and the growth of the specialty. With the advent of microscopic surgery and long complex operations impaired by patient movement, local anesthesia was no longer feasible. It is used infrequently today except for removal of low-grade gliomas in brain areas of language or motor function. In recent years, image guidance and functional MRI improved the preoperative and intra-operative identification of critical areas and pathways, removing some of the unique value of awake functional testing associated with local anesthesia.

Observations while operating on the brain with the patient awake did advance knowledge of brain function in that period between Wilder Penfield beginning in Montreal in 1930 and the advent of sophisticated computer guidance in the '80s. In that era, curious and observant neurosurgeons made multiple, diverse contributions to the knowledge of brain function.

Neurological Imaging – Angiography

In 1961 the three essential elements in a neurosurgical center were the specialty patient care floor, the neurosurgical OR, and neuro-radiology. Images of the blood vessels in the brain (angiography) taken to show the arteries, the intermediate circulation, and the veins were a major element of neuroradiology. Obtaining all of the information required taking multiple pictures as the contrast agent coursed through the vessels of the brain. Initially, we lacked a rapid film changer to provide multiple films. We used a manual pull box that allowed me to take only three films. To plan surgery, we needed to film rapidly to obtain critical information as the contrast agent passed through the circulation.

The Radiology Department was reluctant to ask the hospital leadership to buy a film changer. The radiologists in the department were unconvinced of the value of cerebral angiography and questioned the value of a film changer. After several years, it became apparent that brain surgery was being performed in Peoria and angiography had a critical role in pre-operative evaluation. Radiology asked the hospital to purchase a single plane Sanchez Perez changer costing $2500. The machine shook, the films were not optimum, the changer was slow, and only one plane could be obtained with an injection. Two injections were required to obtain a lateral and AP view, and a third injection if an oblique view was needed. Despite these limitations, we obtained six films with one injection, a vast improvement over the pull box. During this period, momentous technological improvements were occurring in Sweden and Great Britain with radiologists specializing in neuroradiology, and we were woefully behind in the United States and Peoria.

Dr. Robert Wright, one of the early group of American radiologists capable of catheter angiography joined Saint Francis Hospital in 1968. At the same time Dr. William Albers, the University of Illinois pediatric cardiologist, needed a heart catheterization laboratory. With a committed cooperative effort, we obtained a Swedish Elema Schoenander biplane film changer with Siemens three phase radiographic generators to produce the x-rays. In one step, we moved to a state of the art cerebral angiography laboratory in the basement of the central wing of the original hospital building, the only facility of this quality in downstate Illinois. Both cerebral angiography and pediatric heart studies were performed in this room, and we were quite busy from the beginning. With one injection, I could get detailed lateral and AP films of the blood vessels, as the contrast agent passed from arteries to veins. Films could be obtained as rapidly as six per second. An immense amount of additional information was suddenly available. At that time, I told Dr. George Zwicky, one of the senior radiologists, that my ambition was to have more neuroradiology than barium studies in the radiology department. Barium studies were used to study the stomach and colon and created much of the work of the department. This seemingly outrageous change took only ten years.

Dr. Wright was uniquely talented, worked day and night, was always looking for improvement, and we soon were making some of the best angiograms in the United States. Each evening, he formed the catheters for the next day, creating catheter shapes he needed to thread into the various blood vessels to be studied. He placed the needle in the groin, then threaded the fine catheter up through to the vessels leading to the brain with remarkable skill. Since CT and MRI of the brain were not yet invented, detailed study of the arterial and venous anatomy was utilized for brain tumor localization. Dr. Wright's pioneering efforts were largely unsung because we were not publishing the work. He was pioneering percutaneous catheter cerebral angiography in very small children as well. At the time, I visited Dr. Juan Taveras, the Chief of Radiology at the Mallinckrodt Department of Radiology at Washington University in Saint Louis, one of the pioneer neuro-radiologists in the United States. I asked him what technique they used for catheter vertebral angiography in small children, and he assured me "catheter angiography is not feasible in children, too much morbidity". Unfortunately, we were not publishing this work. We just were not cognizant of the importance of publication in medical progress.

Angiography Before Neuroradiologists

Katherine Issac, a 19-year-old college freshman, and daughter of a Peoria internist, was home for spring break. She developed sudden onset of intense headache, was admitted to hospital, and lumbar puncture revealed bloody spinal fluid. She needed cerebral angiography to determine if a ruptured intracranial aneurysm had leaked into the fluid surrounding the brain. That afternoon, she was brought to the radiology department. I inserted an 18 gauge needle in the right common carotid artery in the neck after injecting a local anesthetic, and two injections for an AP and lateral carotid arteriogram revealed a normal study.

I then injected the left carotid artery with 10 CC of contrast agent (35% Diodrast). She immediately could not speak and was unable to move her right arm and leg. Perhaps I had injected the contrast agent into the wall of the artery, closing off the carotid? I feared that dissection in the lining of the carotid artery had occurred. The films were developed, and I reviewed them "wet" in about three minutes, and found that the injection appeared perfect. After 18 of the longest minutes I have ever experienced, she began to speak and over the next 20 minutes, regained all function.

A relatively rare event had occurred, temporary loss of function after injection of this ionic compound that appeared to be irritating to the blood vessels. When injected into the common carotid artery, it always caused facial flushing and pain for perhaps 60 seconds. The left carotid arteriogram was entirely normal as well. With trepidation, the following day, after steroid preparation, I did a brachial angiogram, a technique we were using to fill the vertebrobasilar arteries during the period before catheter angiography, and this too was normal. An aneurysm or arteriovenous malformation was not present. Katherine went on to a full recovery, her illness falling into the category of what we now call a perimesencephalic hemorrhage that generally has an excellent outlook with a very low risk of re-hemorrhage. Contrast agents have steadily improved, and one more risk became history.

From 1961 until Dr. Wright's arrival in 1968, I performed percutaneous cerebral angiography multiple times per week. Angiography was extensively used in the investigation of trauma, tumor, and vascular abnormalities before the advent of CT and MRI imaging. Non-ionic contrast agents coupled with catheter angiography introduced through the groin yielded increasing safety and comfort for patients. The complication rate associated with cerebral angiography in the hands of a talented neuro-radiologist is in the 0.1% range, a formidable improvement over several decades. This day is one of the most memorable in my experience. I was very thankful that I did not have to tell Katherine's father her studies were normal, but my testing caused permanent loss of language function and right arm and leg paralysis.

Air Studies:
Pneumoencephalography and
Ventriculography

Walter Dandy of Johns Hopkins Hospital in 1919, introduced the concept of replacing cerebrospinal fluid in the ventricles of the brain with air to diagnose mass lesions in the brain. This was a major step forward in brain diagnosis that was slowly accepted. Dr. Cushing in Boston resisted the use of air study, probably because Dandy developed the procedure. The long-standing Dandy-Cushing antipathy probably was a factor slowing the utilization of air study in neuroradiology. Introduction of air often made the patient quite ill with a headache, and if they had a brain tumor, induced swelling with acute worsening of the patient's condition. If the air were introduced by direct puncture of the brain and ventricle through a skull opening, and a brain tumor was found, the patient had to be taken directly to surgery, with little time for further study, consultation, and contemplation.

In patients without obvious increased intracranial pressure, the air was introduced via lumbar puncture. This procedure was termed pneumoencephalography. We used a rotating chair to summersault the patient to position the air in the head to obtain the required images. We performed slow turning of the head while the film was exposed, producing an "auto-tomogram". This procedure revealed brain midline structures by blurring out the more peripheral structures that moved enough to obscure them. Introduction and positioning of the air and interpretation of the films was a slowly acquired essential art. In the first ten years in Peoria before CT scanning, ventriculography was the first step in most brain tumor operations.

Older patients were often confused for several days after pneumoencephalography, even when the study did not reveal a tumor or mass lesion. Brain tumor patients often deteriorated neurologically after an air study, in the hours before surgery. After doing the craniotomy and opening the covering of the brain, it was often apparent the air study had increased brain swelling. By the mid-'70s and the advent of CT brain scans, air studies were no longer necessary. The second 20th-century revolution in neurosurgery, computerized imaging, eliminated air studies. My slowly acquired skill needed to place the air in the proper place in the brain and evaluate the images was of no value. Graeme Robertson's classic book on pneumoencephalography became an anachronism. Good riddance! Patients now obtained a diagnosis without an excruciating headache lasting days, or the risks of precipitous worsening of their condition. Neurosurgery was making steady progress.

Myelography

In 1960, tumors, herniated discs, and other problems in the spinal canal were demonstrated by injecting a fat-soluble contrast agent, Pantopaque, into the spinal canal via a lumbar puncture with a large 18 gauge spinal needle. After introduction of the contrast agent, fluoroscopy was done, while the patient was turned and tilted in a dark room, allowing us to observe the spinal canal and take films. The contrast agent was placed into the cervical spine with the head tilted far back to prevent the Pantopaque running into the head, where it could not be retrieved. The prolonged extension of the neck was painful in most patients over 50. Image intensifiers to improve our ability to see the image were not yet available. We walked about with red glasses to allow our eyes to accommodate for an hour or so before the procedure. With accommodation and preparation, images were still indistinct. We obtained multiple spot films, much like a portrait photographer, and awaited the development of these films to make a final diagnosis.

A large gauge needle was used because the oily contrast agent was removed at the end of the procedure. It was believed, that if left in place, the contrast material would produce inflammation and scarring in the subarachnoid space around the brain and spinal cord (arachnoiditis). The aspiration process generated nerve root pain in the leg when a nerve root was sucked against the needle. Since a large needle was used, most patients had a prolonged post-spinal headache, often with vomiting. The spinal fluid continued to leak through the puncture in the dura into the tissues in the back, generating the headache. A painful and trying experience for the patient. Patients rarely permitted a second study.

In the '70s water-soluble agents became available, first in Europe, then the United States. This permitted the use of a smaller gauge needle because the contrast agent was absorbed and did not require removal. Non-ionic Metrizamide was introduced in 1977. In the several years before, studies done by inexperienced staff sometimes resulted in seizures after the ionic water-soluble contrast agent was allowed to escape into the cranial space. The addition of CT to the procedure allowed use of smaller amounts of contrast agent while yielding more precise images. This technique was utilized heavily until spinal MRI scans arrived in the late '80s. Now myelography is rarely necessary. Again, a professional expertise acquired with lengthy experience now became obsolete, with a striking improvement in the patient experience.

Radioisotope Brain Scanning

In the early '60s, air studies and angiography were essential invasive tools for the diagnosis of brain lesions. Radioisotope brain imaging was introduced at the National Hospital, Queen Square, London in 1963. Isotope imaging was rapidly developed at Saint Francis Hospital by Dr. Ben Berg, a pioneer in brain isotope imaging. Isotope studies were immensely helpful in the short period before the availability of computerized tomography. Technetium 99 injected intravenously was taken up by a brain tumor and other lesions. The technique was moderately successful in providing anatomical localization of brain tumor and chronic subdural hematoma, blood clots over the surface of the brain. The deterioration precipitated by air studies was avoided. Non-invasive diagnosis of a brain tumor in a fashion that did not necessitate an immediate trip to the operating room was possible. This utilization of isotopes for tumor diagnosis became obsolete with improving CT scans of the brain in the mid-'70s.

Single Photon Emission Computed Tomography (SPECT) and Positron Emission Tomography (PET) now use isotopes for physiologic studies of blood flow in the brain in some ischemic conditions, and metabolic activity in temporal lobe epilepsy. Determination of biological activity of tumors guides management in some patients, such as those with malignant peripheral neurofibromas. Radioisotope markers are being investigated to study Alzheimer's disease, Parkinson's disease, other degenerative diseases, and mental illness. The potential development of additional biomarkers for degenerative disease has significant research potential. With isotope labeling, specific disease biomarkers can be revealed and we are able to derive brain function information indirectly. Some applications are limited by the short half-life of the study isotope, necessitating an on-site cyclotron. An exciting evolution in technology from rather crudely demonstrating anatomical information in the '60s to eloquently displaying physiology, metabolism, and brain function in the current era.

The First Brain Tumor

Mr. Fritz Ziegler, a 56-year-old manager at the Hiram Walker

Distillery, was referred because of difficulty lifting his right foot. His physician thought he had a pinched nerve in his lower back causing a "drop foot." When I watched him walk he lifted the foot higher to step and tripped at times. He did not swing his right arm as he did his left. I reviewed his x-rays before examining him and, indeed, he did have narrowing of his L4 disc with some arthritic change, the reason for the referral. On examination, his reflexes were abnormally brisk in the right arm and right leg, and he had an up going great toe with plantar stimulation of the right foot, a Babinski sign. These signs indicated the problem was in the brain, not the lumbar spine. Initial weakness in the right foot suggested a benign tumor growing from the covering of the brain near the midline, a parasagittal meningioma. The brain responsible for foot movement is near the midline at the top of the brain. The ability to learn so much from the history and examination of the patient was the great attraction of neurology.

In 1961, before isotope brain scanning or CT, the next step was angiography to detect characteristic abnormal blood vessels seen in a tumor. Fritz was admitted to the hospital, and I performed a percutaneous left carotid arteriogram the next day. I placed a needle in the left carotid artery in the neck after palpating the artery and threaded the needle up the artery a bit. We did not have film changers, so a box containing three films was used with the technician rapidly pulling each film cassette obtaining three images as the contrast agent went through the brain. I called "shoot" after I had injected half of the contrast agent, and injected the remaining 4cc. A lateral view was obtained. The x-ray tube was then changed and a frontal or AP view was obtained in a similar fashion. The needle was removed, pressure maintained on the artery for ten minutes, and the developed films were reviewed. I inspected the films while they were "wet", the developing process not entirely completed. These revealed a classic meningioma stain produced by abnormal dural arteries filling the tumor in the left parasagittal region. My suspicions were confirmed. The patient was scheduled for surgery the following day.

In December 1961, the patient's head was held in place on the OR table with small sandbags and tape after positioning. After shaving the entire head, I outlined the appropriate incision. The scalp was cleansed with alcohol and bichloride of mercury just as Harvey Cushing had done in Boston in 1930. I then turned down a scalp flap and made six holes with a Cushing perforator followed by an enlarging burr. These instruments were designed to minimize the danger of plunging into the brain. Each hole was then connected with the Gigli saw, essentially a flexible braided wire with small teeth to cut the bone. This process involved a great deal of physical work and about 60 minutes to complete.

After lifting the bone flap, the dura with the enlarged blood vessels and the underlying tumor was apparent. We were in the correct position on the appropriate side of the head. I opened the dura and sealed each of the larger blood vessels with a Cushing silver clip. At this point, I donned my headlight with its electric lamp, and Keeler loupes, and dissected the tumor away from the brain, using multiple pledgets of cotton. A significant portion of dura was involved in the tumor, so I made an incision over the left hip and took a graft of fascia lata (the fibrous covering of the muscle) and repaired the covering of the brain, sutured it with fine silk, and wired the bone flap in place. The scalp was closed in two layers, galea, and skin, the skin with millinery needles in Dr. Cushing's style. A large head dressing was applied, and the patient returned to the recovery room then to his room on the orthopedic floor. The operation was little changed from Dr. Cushing's method at the Brigham Hospital in Boston in 1930 except the diagnosis was made with angiography rather than air study. Identification of this precise localization permitted a smaller skull opening than in Cushing's era.

Fritz made a rapid and uneventful recovery and was walking

normally in ten days after a one-week hospital stay. An effective head holder, air driven instruments for bone work, bipolar cautery forceps, and surgical microscope would all come a decade later. Despite these technical limitations, a curative resection without complication was readily accomplished. The brain surgery practice had begun.

Medulloblastoma: Failure at Christmas

Sue Peterson, the first child with a brain tumor I saw in Peoria, was four years old and was admitted after two weeks of persistent vomiting. She was the only child of young parents who were the ministers of a small church and settlement house on the near north side of Peoria. Sue had straw-colored hair, blue eyes, a winsome smile, and held her doll tightly for security. On examination, she had papilledema (swelling of the optic nerve discs) in both eyes, an indication of increased intracranial pressure. Her walk was a little unsteady, but all other functions were intact.

She was admitted to the children's floor, and the next day, I did a ventriculogram, introducing air in the ventricles, revealing hydrocephalous and obstruction of the 4th ventricle in the base of the brain. In her age group, this indicated a probable medulloblastoma, the common malignant brain tumor of childhood located in the base of the brain in the cerebellum. The benign tumor, a piloid astrocytoma, unfortunately, was less likely. She was returned to the operating room, and I removed the tumor seemingly completely from the midline of the cerebellum. This was done with a headlight and my Keeler surgical loupes and required two and a half hours. She awakened promptly in the recovery room, and made a miraculous recovery. Pathology of the frozen tumor sections revealed the dreaded medulloblastoma.

Sitting with the parents later that day, I had to tell them that the life expectancy was only a year or two and none of these tumors were cured. They found this difficult to believe because she seemed well in all other respects. Afterward, radiation treatments were administered daily for almost a month. She did not eat well, lost her hair, then began to improve and seemed normal. Her mother and father were certain that I was mistaken about her outlook.

She did well until early December a year later when her symptoms returned and became worse rapidly. The parents and I decided to keep her at home, and she gradually went into coma. I made a house call to see her in the late evening, on Christmas eve, in Averyville in North Peoria and spent a long time with her mother and father. I walked out of the house at midnight. There was a full moon, a crisp night and the saddest feeling of my life, before or since. Sue's parents remained in Peoria and continued a program dedicated to supporting the poor of the North end.

In subsequent years, the treatment of medulloblastoma has become much better, with chemotherapy and improved radiation, allowing some patients to be cured and others living at least three to five years. Some of the surviving patients have a diminution of higher brain function secondary to radiation and chemotherapy resulting in school difficulties and occupational limitations. Research continues to drive relentless progress in malignant childhood tumors, a much more hopeful future than experienced that Christmas Eve, so long ago.

A Permanent Roof over Our Head

After a year in Peoria, our daughter Katherine was born, and the tiny apartment was not a place to raise a family. My dream of living in the country disappeared, destroyed by endless calls to the emergency room every night, sometimes followed by all night surgery. Living near the hospital was imperative. While Gladys and Katherine were in the hospital, I looked at houses, finding a large, old home on Moss Avenue in the Bradley University neighborhood. It was 5 minutes from the hospital, with a large tree filled lot and a house some distance from the street.

After considering the matter for six months, we decided to purchase. The house was still available, the neighborhood, at the time deemed undesirable because it was "inner city". We were totally naïve, and unqualified to evaluate real estate. We moved from a tiny apartment to a two-story 50-year-old house with multiple rooms in one faith-based leap. We spent 55 years repairing it and appreciating the effort Mr. Martin Seine expended in building a detail-filled house in 1915. There is a long screened porch across the back of the house, with an old-fashioned swing that accommodates a man taller than me, stretched out for leisurely summer reading. The one acre backyard provided a venue for all the gardening a person desires. The three car garage is 300 feet downhill from the house and fully equipped for charging a 1918 electric car, but ill adapted to modern lifestyle and Midwestern winters.

In the ensuing four years, two sons, Eric and John arrived and the house seemed filled with children. The opportunity to raise the family in the inner city with an inner city school experience was a sound decision. I was able to return to the hospital when worried about a patient, yet have dinner with the family every evening. This could not have been achieved in the suburbs or metropolitan center — Country brain surgery had advantages!

Katherine began school at Whittier Grade School in the neighborhood and then transferred to Washington School four blocks down Moss Avenue, and both boys followed. The children walked to school on sidewalks; a non-suburban childhood.

The neighborhood cohesiveness added to the quality of life by supporting neighborhood activities and Westminster Presbyterian and Saint Mark's Church. Sidewalks were filled with walkers and runners before either was fashionable. Katherine, Eric, and John were able to take music and other lessons on the Bradley University campus, a short walk from home. It was an idyllic small town existence.

Consultations Away from the Center

I walked into the room, and the special duty nurse turned and said: "doctor, I believe the patient just passed away". I received a call from a physician in Macomb, Illinois four hours earlier. He asked me to drive over and see a 37-year-old man admitted the previous day with an intense headache and drowsiness. The patient had become steadily more drowsy overnight. That morning, a lumbar puncture revealed bloody spinal fluid, indicating bleeding into the fluid around the brain, and no evidence of infection.

In 1961, patients were rarely transferred from outlying hospitals without a prior consultative visit. I told the doctor I was concerned about a possible brain aneurysm as the cause of the subarachnoid hemorrhage and the patient needed to be transferred for angiography. He asked me to come to see the patient in consultation. I started to Macomb in my new Volkswagen Beetle, a 2-hour drive on two-lane rural roads. On arrival, the referring physician immediately met me and we proceeded to the room. In that era, there were no intensive care beds, and critically ill patients often had special duty nurses that were assigned from a hospital roster. The special duty nurses usually did not have extensive knowledge of the problem and were often less informed than the staff floor nurses.

I rapidly examined the patient; he had died, after deteriorating in the preceding several hours. A ruptured brain aneurysm was the probable cause, and his doctor and I talked with the family. They were understandably in turmoil and to better understand what had happened wished to have an autopsy. I remained in Macomb and assisted the hospital pathologist with the autopsy.

The cause of the brain hemorrhage was an anterior communicating aneurysm deep in the middle of the brain. This information helped his wife and parents better understand the tragedy.

Twenty or more hospitals from 30 to 130 miles away referred patients to Saint Francis, and the transfer was done by local ambulance services. Evaluation of the patient's condition before the transfer was difficult because x-rays and medical records were not available for review. Physicians often requested I come and see the patient in consultation before committing to a transfer. The immediate result was long trips at the end of the day to see consultations in hospitals that ranged in size for 20 beds to 150 beds with variable facilities. I took a set of surgical instruments in the car at times, because emergency surgery was expected at some of the larger hospitals for an open head injury or an intracranial hematoma. It is often said today that American medical care is not a system, and in the '60s that was unequivocally true.

The Vietnam War bought a new era with expertise in helicopter evacuation and trauma centers. Saint Francis was a leader in downstate Illinois with the early development of a Level 1 Trauma center. Dr. Stuart Roberts, who served as a leading surgeon in Vietnam, came to Peoria and began a program to bring helicopter transfer to Peoria. The first helicopter transfer was a premature baby transferred in the Peoria Journal Star newspaper helicopter on January 10, 1967. The helicopter had two seats and could only transfer premature infants.

Later in the '70s, the Illinois Department of Transportation assumed the role of transferring critically ill in their Bell 206 Jet Rangers. The SFMC Life Flight was organized in 1984 and initially used a Bell Long Ranger provided by the Illinois Department of Transportation (IDOT). It was often unavailable, and SFMC leased their first helicopter in October 1986. The program continued to grow. A fleet of four American Eurocopter EC 145 helicopters and a Hanger dedicated to Dr. Stuart Roberts now serves over thirty hospitals in Illinois. This was a long transition from military wound management transportation to civilian transport to a clinical center. Historically war has often contributed significantly to the advancement of medical care, and it of interest that the lessons learned in Vietnam regarding transportation of the ill took so long to be implemented in civilian life.

Years later, we developed a system-wide x-ray imaging system allowing review of films taken at any OSF hospital (PACS). We then added an additional system to download images into our servers from other referring hospitals. The immediate result was an ability to assess thoroughly the patients in outlying facilities. The availability of rapid transport eliminated my long distance traveling consultations. Patients in less populated rural areas now arrived at an appropriate treatment site promptly. Telemedicine technology continues to improve our ability to evaluate at a distance. Clinicians are challenged to change their behavior at the pace of technology change. Obsolescence is easily achieved!

Diving Disasters: Labor Day 1961

By Labor Day of the first year in Peoria, a daily routine for clinic and surgery was established. Dr. Holden was flying to upstate New York for the Labor Day holiday. The weather was beautiful, and the emergency rooms were full. On Saturday afternoon, I was called by the Saint Francis Emergency Room to care for Eric Trent, a 17-year-old boy who had arrived unable to move his arms and legs after diving in their farm pond. I went to the hospital immediately. On examination, Eric could only flex his elbows, and there was absence of feeling below the thumbs in his hands bilaterally, indicating probable complete loss of spinal cord function below the C5-6 level.

A portable x-ray revealed a partially collapsed 6th cervical vertebrae in the neck with a forward movement of the 5th vertebrae on the 6th. This produced a profound narrowing of the spinal canal and damaged the spinal cord. The spine had to be stabilized and alignment established before he could be moved. I numbed his scalp and with a small drill placed a drill hole halfway through the skull on each side in the parietal region and attached a Crutchfield skull tong, connecting it to 25 pounds of weight to gradually realign the vertebrae with traction. Eric was placed on a Stryker frame bed, a special device that allowed us to turn him from front to back every two hours without displacing his neck.

At the time, this was state-of-the-art treatment. Virtually all were permanent injuries, leaving the patient unable to walk or effectively use their arms with loss of bowel and bladder control. The worst conceivable accident in a boy's life. Since pre-hospital field care treatment was not well developed, virtually all patients arrived with a "complete" injury, a transection of the spinal cord at the level of injury. If the original injury did not completely damage the spinal cord, moving the patient to the hospital often completed the injury. The patients were maintained in traction for 6-12 weeks, then placed in a brace or cast for a period, while they were gradually transitioned to a wheelchair. Relatively few patients had a fusion procedure done at that time unless the dislocation could not be reduced.

After the initial examination, I came out and talked with his father, discussing the ominous outlook. He was a massive man, at least six inches taller than me, wearing bib overalls. He looked at me, and said: "you ain't old enough to take care of my boy." At the time, I was 28 years old with a crew haircut and probably looked like a high school boy to the father. Dr. Holden was away, I informed him I was all he had till Tuesday, and he accepted that. By Tuesday, having aged perhaps ten years that weekend, I was old enough.

Sunday and Monday saw more accidents with spinal cord injury; Monday night there were three quadriplegic patients in tong traction on the orthopedic floor. I had used all of the Crutch-field tongs in the city and urgently ordered two sets Tuesday morning from Codman and Shurtleff, the leading neurosurgical instrument firm.

Most of the injuries occurred in young men 15-25 who were diving in shallow water, driving an automobile, or riding a motor-cycle. The problem was always a foreign concept to patient and family. I came to the hospital at night frequently to see them at times of anxiety and fright, both on the part of the patients, the families, and the inexperienced nurses struggling to care for them. In that era, it was an emotionally draining part of neuro-surgical practice experienced by most active neurosurgeons who were not part of a University teaching program. In the teaching programs, the residents bore the brunt of the emotional relation-ships although the faculty was ultimately responsible for care.

At that time, Dr. Ralph Cloward in Hawaii advocated ante-rior cervical fusion and presented a paper in 1958 to the Harvey Cushing Society. Dr. Cloward felt he could avoid the prolonged traction and begin early ambulation with this fusion. His work was initially treated with derision and disdain by established neuro-surgery. He persisted, steadily improving the instrumentation, and organized neurosurgery slowly adapted and improved the techniques. Cloward's technique has been replaced by improved technology. He was a major contributor to the anterior approach to the spine. Over several years, anterior and posterior fusion techniques developed, and long periods in traction and bed rest were avoided. The advent of trauma systems resulted in safer extraction and transfer of patients with spinal injury. Additional injury rarely occurs in transport and patients now often arrive with incomplete spinal injury rather than complete transection of the spinal cord so prevalent in the 60's.

It was not until 1986 that the neurosurgical organizations began Think First, a national education program in primary and secondary schools to prevent spinal injuries. Neurosurgery as a profession was slow to accept responsibility for prevention programs; instead focusing entirely on their limited hospital role. These preventive programs and trauma management have reduced the frequency of these tragedies in the young. Unfortunately, more recently with aging in America, we care for people in their '80s and '90s who have injured their spinal cord in a fall, something quite rare 50 years ago.

Peoria was a pioneer in rehabilitation, led by Dr. Worley Kendall. Worley arrived in Peoria from the Institute for Rehabilitation Medicine in New York, the first rehabilitation facility in the United States. This development in Peoria was supported by the Sommer Family's Forest Park Foundation, demonstrating an amazing early insight for this societal need. The four-story Forest Park Rehabilitation Institute was located across Glen Oak Avenue from Saint Francis Hospital. Patients with spinal cord injury from around the state were transferred for further care. In 1961, we provided state-of-the-art rehabilitation in a small Midwestern town. The persistence of the Sommer family and their Forest Park Foundation created a unique facility. A physical medicine and rehabilitation residency program trained physician specialists in the new field. Upon Dr. Kendall's retirement, the Institute lost momentum and the residency training program closed. Dr. Kendall demonstrated the difference so often made by one person. Unfortunately, he also demonstrated that improvement is tenuous, if an enduring infrastructure is not created.

The lack of progress in spinal injury care from the '50s to the '80s is troublesome. Organized medicine and neurosurgery were slow to address prevention with education, seat belts, and facility redesign. Neurological surgery did not address spinal biomechanics and stability. Orthopedic surgery pioneered operations to stabilize the spine, and neurosurgery followed. Orthopedists were experienced in rehabilitation after their work with polio patients.

Finally, neurosurgery was tardy in the development of rehabilitation, orthotics, and robotics to aid the disabled. Looking back at this process in 2018, neurosurgery lacked direction and leadership through that period. There is a lesson in this process: What are the important problems in society and are we addressing them as a profession? Our departmental and specialty leadership did not ask the right questions then and are we asking them now? In research, framing the questions is crucial; this is just as critical in clinical medicine. Critical questioners remain in short supply.

The Neurosurgery Board Examination: The Final Step

American specialty medicine rapidly evolved in the early '50s; formal residency specialty training programs were established and certification by specialty board examination became a critical career milestone. The American Board of Neurological Surgery (ABNS) was formed in Chicago in 1940, and Dr. Oldberg participated in the development. The ABNS was formed late, the American Board of Ophthalmology was created in 1916 and the American Board of Psychiatry and Neurology (ABPN) had been in place since 1934. In the early '60s, there were still many non-certified practicing neurosurgeons, but the expectation for certification was clear.

Two years of clinical work after residency was required before one could sit for the oral examination of the American Board of Neurological Surgery. I was swamped by clinical work, procrastinated, and delayed collecting my year of required case records. Because of the delay in application, my examination was in April 1964, almost three years after finishing the residency. During that three year interval, I worked seven days a week, skipped national meetings, but did read the current literature carefully. I avoided formal preparation for the examination and did not talk with others who had taken the Boards. Before the appointed day, I drove to Chicago and studied one full day before the oral examination. I obtained a motel room in Evanston and read neurophysiology, my greatest weakness, for 12 hours.

On the appointed day, I went to the Neuropsychiatric Institute at the University of Illinois, arriving 30 minutes early. The oral examination was given from its inception in the offices on the 5th and 6th floors of the NPI. The hall was filled with candidates milling around and asking "where is Elwood?" This, of course, caused anxiety, but it was soon apparent that there was one unplanned candidate, and the examiners simply wanted me to start early. I had trained at the NPI and knew where to go without instruction.

Fifty-four years later most details of the day are obscure, but some vivid memories remain. There were six oral examinations: neurosurgery, neurology, neuroradiology, general surgery, neuropathology, and neuroanatomy-neurophysiology. Each subject had two examiners. One examiner was a member of the board, and the other a visiting expert in the topic of the specific examination.

I waited outside the door of the neuroradiology examination, my first examination, because they were running over with their candidate. Finally, the door opened. The candidate stepped out, looking very pale and near collapse. Dr. Mayfield beckoned me in. Things seemed ominous! Two neurosurgeons conducted the neuroradiology examination. This was indicative of the state of the art of neuroradiology in the United States, at that time. Neuroradiology as a specialty had hardly begun, neurosurgeons were the experts. I answered the first two questions to their satisfaction, and they then provided some esoteric problems to test my limits. All went well, and I left the room ready to tackle the remaining examiners.

In Neurosurgery, Dr. Colin McCarty, the Chief at the Mayo

Clinic was my principal examiner. His questions required specific operative experience that fortunately reflected my surgical series. In neuropathology, although Dr. Orville Bailey had been my professor, he and a neurosurgeon examined me. The other neurosurgeon assured objectivity and Dr. Bailey was the only neuropathologist available.

The real fright came in neuroanatomy and neurophysiology. I opened the door to see Dr. Stephan Gurdjian as the primary examiner. He was the chief of neurosurgery in Detroit, had a Ph.D. in neurophysiology, and was an expert in diencephalic and thalamic anatomy and physiology. He began to explore that physiology with me, promptly put his finger on my weaknesses and examined them further in a gentle but probing fashion. At this point, I felt uncertain about the outcome of this process, perhaps 12 hours of neurophysiology study was inadequate.

The board met at the end of the examination, and after a two-hour wait, each candidate was called to receive their result at a long table in the library of the NPI. The secretary of the Board, Dr. Donald Matson gave the pass or fail verdict with no prolonged waiting for a letter! Dr. Matson smiled, said I passed, and I returned to Peoria that night elated. This was my first exposure to Don Matson, who was remarkably cordial and kind while delivering the potentially life-altering verdict to the candidates. At the time, he was developing pediatric neurosurgery as a specialty at the Children's Hospital in Boston. Sadly, he died of Creutzfeldt-Jakob Disease (a rapidly fatal degenerative brain disease caused by a prion), in 1969 at age fifty-six, five years after my first meeting with him in Chicago. He had been exposed to this prion disease with a needle stick while doing a brain biopsy on a patient with the disease.

Dr. Oldberg, several weeks later, informed me that Colin McCarty, President of the Board, had called him to say that my performance on the oral had been excellent. The days study in

Evanston had saved me from failure with Dr. Gurdjian.

Neurosurgery residency programs varied a great deal in quality in the '50s, with some mediocre programs and disregard for pedagogy principles. The failure rate in the oral examination was unacceptably high. The Board developed a written examination as a prerequisite to oral examination to assess cognitive competence. The oral examination then became a final step in board certification after two years of clinical practice and successful completion of the written examination. The pass rate improved immediately because candidates generally arrived with an adequate cognitive base.

I was now certified as a competent neurosurgeon for the rest of my life, no more examinations, at least not in medicine! This clearly was not an acceptable state in a rapidly changing field. In 1985, the decision was made to issue the certificate for ten years, with maintenance of certification required. The recertification examination process would continue for life, reflecting the need for lifelong learning in a field that significantly changes every 5-to-10 years.

In 1983, I was a guest examiner at the Board Examination in New Orleans. Because the written examination did much of the evaluation of the cognitive base, the oral examination consisted of three one-hour examinations: cranial, spinal, and neurology with two examiners in each session. The pass rate had improved to 85 percent, and the emphasis was on safe practice and less on minute factual detail.

Some of the candidates came poorly prepared for the examination. On my return to Peoria, I developed a yearly oral examination for our residents to improve their preparation for the certification process. I served as a guest examiner in Houston in 1992 and in Baltimore in 1999, each time acquiring insights to enhance our annual resident oral examination and the residency experience.

With certification, I was eligible for admission to the Harvey

Cushing Society, becoming a member in 1967. Later that year, the Society name was changed to the American Association of Neurological Surgeons, reflecting the fact that the majority of American neurosurgeons no longer had any relationship to the Cushing lineage. My teachers, Dr. Eric Oldberg and Dr. Percival Bailey, had been so involved with Cushing at the Brigham that I had an emotional attachment to the "Harvey Cushing Society". Although the Harvey Cushing Society name no longer fitted the mission, some of our history was lost with the name change.

Medicare and "Socialized Medicine" 1965

A revolution in the economics of medical care began in 1965. In Peoria, Caterpillar was the major employer, and their employee insurance plan provided economic stability in the medical community. The maximum surgical fee $250, was paid for a craniotomy. Patients usually were unable to pay anything in addition to the insurance fee. Most people retired at 65, and many were already disabled or unable to work. The physicians in the community cared for people over 65 receiving little compensation because older people simply were unable to pay physicians or hospitals. Many children were not covered by an insurance plan. Some help was provided by the Division of Services for Crippled Children to children with neurosurgical problems. I believe about 30 percent of care by physicians and hospitals, in 1965, was uncompensated, an unsustainable economic model.

Physicians were resistant to Medicare and Medicaid programs, assuming these programs were the beginning of socialized medicine similar to that of post WW II Britain. They were aware and sympathetic to the stresses that older patients experienced and cared for them without payment. They were more concerned about infringement on their independence than the economic stability of a health care system.

Medicare and Medicaid programs were signed into law by President Lyndon Johnson on July 30, 1965, and the medical world did not end. Physicians and hospitals began to receive small fees for the care of the elderly and medical practice changed little. The fear of medical bankruptcy decreased in the elderly, and they were less reluctant to seek medical care. In the past 50 years, the program has evolved, still has many imperfections and inefficiencies, but has provided much-appreciated peace of mind to the elderly who previously approached all medical care with fear of dreadful impoverishment.

At the time, an all-consuming daily workload obliterated my awareness of politics and economics. Clearly Medicare legislation was a necessary step, first broached by President Truman, and accomplished by President Johnson and now an essential element of the American fabric. I believe the take-home message is that it is imperative those in medicine be attuned to the suffering and pain of our general society. Although we have arrived at a point where we now utilize a substantial part of the GDP (17.3%), patients generally have better health care than their parents, and function well until late in life as the result of expensive joint replacements, coronary stents, and other complex, expensive care.

As our contribution to the social contract, we are obliged to make medical care better and less expensive through process improvement achieved by competitive American industries. This requires an entrepreneurial attitude and mind set of someone in the San Francisco Bay Area rather than an entitlement approach to the status quo. There is an urgency for this culture change.

Medicare, although disparaged as a government program, has lower overhead than the multiple private insurance plans in the United States. The legislation explicitly forbids the Medicare administration to develop a highly competitive medication pricing program, as established in European health plans. Competitive pricing of medication, implants, and supplies, and avoidance of treatments that have not been proven to be effective have potential for substantial improvement in the fiscal viability of the Medicare program.

The Dartmouth data (Dartmouth Atlas of Health Care) continues to highlight striking differences in the utilization of tests, procedures and surgical operations in different population areas in the United States demonstrating a potential for improvement in use of resources. This data has shown twice as many cardiac catheterization and cardiac stenting and surgery performed in one south Texas community as in a nearby small city with similar population characteristics.

An important part of the Medicare legislation added in 1985 was direct and indirect funding to hospitals for graduate training in medicine, critical funding for training of future medical manpower. An attempt to control the cost of graduate education resulted in a cap on the number of residents, fixing the number of positions to those in place December 31, 1996. The growth of new programs and increase in the size of established programs has thus been limited the past 20 years. Each year, the federal government pays $9.5 billion Medicare dollars to fund graduate education. About $3 billion is spent in direct payments to support salaries of residents and faculty, and $6.5 billion is spent in indirect payments for associated costs of education in hospitals and clinics.

During the subsequent 19-year period, many new allopathic and osteopathic medical schools were created and established schools enlarged their classes, increasing the output of medical schools without providing a corresponding increase in graduate positions. During the same era, there has been a sustained trend to ambulatory care, making hospital oriented graduate education programs less appropriate, in some specialties. The current state requires change in the next five years to assure production of the appropriate medical manpower for the American people, after years of minor temporizing adjustments. We are not prepared for the 50-year Medicare birthday party.

An Eye Surgeon with Hand Weakness

Dr. Henry Clark called at 6:00 a.m., Monday morning, realizing I would be starting rounds at the Proctor Hospital. Henry was the senior ophthalmologist in the city, an excellent cataract surgeon who had pioneered the placement of an intraocular lens, after cataract extraction, in our community. Pain in his neck and left shoulder developed Sunday morning with pain radiating into his arm later in the day. During the night, numbness in the 4th and 5th fingers developed and he felt he could not use his left hand well, a source of concern because he was left-handed. By 1:00 a.m., the pain in the shoulder and arm was excruciating and he could not sleep or lie down. He could get comfortable by standing with both arms elevated on his dresser. Henry spent the night in that position, reluctant to call me till morning.

I saw him immediately at his home, and he was still in severe pain. Examination revealed decreased sensation in the 4th and 5th fingers and the outer part of his hand, and loss of strength in the small muscles of the hand, critical for the work of an eye surgeon. Henry had compression of the C8 nerve root, as it connected to the spinal cord, probably by a fragment of disc material that had ruptured from the disc between the C7 and the T1 vertebrae in the base of the neck. I arranged hospitalization immediately at the Methodist Hospital where he worked. A myelogram that afternoon revealed the expected C7-T1 disc herniation. Surgery was planned for the next morning.

At the time, an acute disc herniation in the neck was operated either from the back of the neck or the front, almost in equal numbers in the United States determined by the training and prior experience of the neurosurgeon. I planned a posterior hemilaminectomy approach. After he was anesthetized, we turned Henry on his abdomen with chest supported and head in a horse-shoe headrest. I made a short incision in the midline over the C7 vertebrae. In most patients, we localized the surgical site by the length of the vertebral spinous process. I drilled out the roof of the spinal canal at the junction of C7 and T1 using a high-speed drill driven by compressed air. This allowed delicate removal of the bone over the nerve without further pinching of this badly compressed nerve. The drill had a variety of tiny burrs that permitted precise exposure.

This drill was a major improvement over the equipment available on my arrival in 1961. Then, I used a low-speed dental drill driven by a thin belt that was difficult to bring into the surgical field. Because of the low speed and dull burrs, the drill had a frightening tendency to skip, at times when one was drilling next to the spinal cord. The new drill made the operation less frightening. I gently moved the nerve, and removed three tiny fragments of broken disc. I closed the incision, the surgery had taken 90 minutes.

Henry was pain-free in the recovery room, the post-operative incisional pain trivial in contrast to the intense pain experienced before surgery. He was walking that evening and insisted on returning home the following day. A full schedule of cataract surgery was possible in two weeks with essentially normal hand function. Operations for herniated cervical disc were technically gratifying because the instrumentation allowed a precise, controlled operation, and the patient relief was often immediate. This balanced, to some extent, the emotional drain of operating on young people with malignant brain tumors and failure to cure or improve their problem.

Part of a Medical Community

After finishing surgery on a summer afternoon in 1962, I was paged on the overhead system by the Proctor Hospital operator as I made rounds. Dr. Harry Adams, a young general surgeon who had been in Peoria 3 years longer than I, was holding on the phone. Harry said he was in surgery at Saint Francis Hospital and had a problem. He was doing a radical mastectomy for breast cancer. In that era, a biopsy was done, and if the tumor was malignant, a radical mastectomy followed without awakening the patient, a process that thankfully has passed into medical history.

Harry was well along in the surgery, had virtually removed the specimen, including the breast tissue, the pectoralis muscle, and the axillary lymph nodes when he realized he had cut a nerve. He was uncertain which nerve had been transected, and was quite worried. I told him I would come immediately, and parked in front of the hospital, at the front door, as luck allowed. Harry was at the front door, awaiting my arrival, and took me directly to the operating room.

At that time, I felt most competent in brain tumor surgery and was less comfortable with the finer points of peripheral nerve repair. Fortunately, I had a sound book knowledge regarding the anatomy. Inspection of the surgical field revealed the nerve involved was the medial cutaneous nerve of the arm, a sensory nerve that would not cause paralysis. Both nerve ends were found, and I sutured them using surgical loupe magnification. Harry and I anxiously awaited the patient's awakening. My examination revealed only a small area of decreased sensation without discernible paralysis. My anatomical assessment was correct. The sensory loss gradually improved over the next year.

Over the years, I was called to the operating room from time to time, after the surgeon found something unexpected or had a complication in process. I have had an opportunity to help, while at times requiring similar aid myself. Support by colleagues occurs in all medical centers and was easily accomplished and comforting in the small cohesive medical center atmosphere experienced in the '60s.

In that era, virtually everyone worked at the three hospitals creating a small, highly supportive medical community. In recent years, most physicians are employed by health care systems, and work in a single institution, resulting in a less collegial medical community. Direct communication has decreased as well, increasing the risk of error. In earlier years, a physician called a consultant, gave the background, and framed the question. The consultant discussed the problem with the referring physician, after his visit, providing an opportunity to assure understanding. Now, consultation requests are entered in the electronic medical record, and the quality of professional interaction has diminished. We are becoming more aware of the danger of diminished communication and must solve the problem. With cell phones and texting, it has never been easier to communicate directly, yet the quality of this communication has decreased in the past ten years, while the need for error-free hand-off has increased exponentially.

Formation of the Neurological Associates

In 1968, around-the-clock work, all-day Saturday surgery, and Sundays' filled with consultations became untenable. I decided to develop a larger neurological group called The Neurological Associates. Larry Holden and I worked well together in our informal relationship, but a sizeable collegial group of neurologists and neurosurgeons was needed to serve our community. I made a trip to Fargo, North Dakota in November 1968 to visit Dr. Christopherson who had established a neurology and neurosurgery group in Fargo to serve North Dakota and Northern Minnesota, a situation very like Peoria. They had three neurosurgeons and three neurologists and were salaried much like the Mayo Clinic where they trained. This encouraged the referral of patients among the staff based on patient requirements, and the neurologists saw most of the medical neurology problems. Their model seemed applicable to Peoria. I returned and asked Larry to join me as a first step in developing a similar group.

Dr. Dennis Garwacki interned at Saint Francis Hospital, after graduating from Northwestern Medical School, and was completing a neurology residency at Wayne State University in Detroit. Dennis liked Peoria, and since he was a Chicago native, was interested in joining us. We had taken the first step in the creation of a combined neurology and neurosurgery practice.

The possible establishment of a downstate branch of the University of Illinois College of Medicine in Peoria was in active discussion, as we formed The Neurological Associates. We installed a neurological library and prepared to create a faculty serving the medical school.

Dr. John Henderson, another Chicagoan, was an intern on my service and found he liked neurosurgery. Jack did his preliminary general surgery residency with us, and we arranged a neurosurgery residency with Dr. Oldberg at the University of Illinois. In July 1971, Dr. Henderson returned to Peoria, joining our new group. Before his arrival, I was available at all times and now alternated with Dr. Henderson, a much-needed change in life- style. Dr. Holden encouraged further development and was an invaluable support, as we began to perform complex operations.

Relatively early Dr. John McLean, who had trained in neurology with Dr. Henderson at Rush Presbyterian, joined Dr. Garwacki in neurology. In 1977, after a lengthy search process, Dr. William Hanigan was recruited to neurosurgery. Bill knew Dr. Lee in Chicago's south side and successfully recruited him to join us. Dr. Richard Lee, who had become familiar with Peoria during an internship at Saint Francis Hospital, contributed epilepsy expertise after completing his neurology residency and EEG fellowship at Northwestern University. Dr. Gaylord Bennett brought expertise in pediatric neurology from the University of Utah, and the clinical neuroscience faculty was growing. Recruitment of specialists who did not have some personal relationship remained difficult. Neurologists and neurosurgeons still wished to stay in established academic centers. Dr. Richard Lister, our first medical student interested in neurosurgery, returned to The Neurological Associates in 1980 after neurosurgery residency at the University of Florida. Twenty years after my arrival in Peoria, a faculty to support an undergraduate and graduate program in neuroscience was finally in place.

The Saga of Hydrocephalus Shunting

An 11 p.m. call from parents of a four-year-old girl living in a small community 100 miles north of Peoria awakened me, after a long day in the operating room. Their daughter Bridget complained of a headache since mid-afternoon, vomited several times, and now was drowsy. I told her mother I would meet them in the Saint Francis Hospital Emergency Room and expected they would arrive shortly after midnight.

I originally cared for Bridget, the first child of young parents, two years before when she first experienced similar symptoms for almost a month. At that time, I found a pretty two-year-old, blond girl who was normal in all respects except for headaches and vomiting. On looking in her eyes, I found papilledema or swelling of the optic nerve, indicating increased pressure in the brain. An air study revealed hydrocephalus with large fluid-filled ventricles. The cause was acqueductal stenosis, a congenital condition narrowing the passage between the third and fourth ventricles of the brain. This narrowing disturbed the flow of cerebrospinal fluid with a secondary fluid buildup in the lateral ventricles and pressure in her brain.

I placed a Pudenz ventriculoatrial shunt, a fine spaghetti-like tube that carried the fluid from the ventricle in the brain to the right atrium of the heart. This involved making a small hole in the skull, threading the fine silastic tube into the ventricle, connecting it to a small flush valve, then through a small incision in the neck, threading the tube into the right atrium of the heart through the jugular vein in the neck. A simple, short operation resulted in Bridget feeling normal in several days, and she returned home, a seeming miracle with great parental relief.

The miracle frequently was not enduring. The fine tubing could be plugged in the brain by the choroid plexus, a fine blood vessel network that floated like seaweed in the ventricle. The choroid was sometimes sucked into the tube, plugging it. Protein and cell collections at times plugged the flush valve or the slit valve at the end of the tubing in the heart. Since this was a foreign object implanted in important structures, the brain and the heart, there was always potential for infection. Development of a cerebrospinal fluid shunt in the late '50s was a miracle for children with hydrocephalus, but an imperfect miracle.

Despite all of these hazards, Bridget did well when I visited with her in the office the following year. She was developing into a bright, energetic little girl. This night, she arrived at Saint Francis Hospital at 1:30 a.m., and the flush valve did not spring up when pumped. This suggested that the top end of the shunt system was plugged in the ventricle. I took her to the operating room and opened the incision over the flush valve, taking a sample for culture for possible infection, and tested the catheter to the heart. It opened at 8 cm of water, as it should; the problem was in the ventricular tubing. The tubing in the heart was fine and did not have to be changed.

I gently pulled the plugged ventricular tubing, and fortunately, it came away readily. At times, the ventricular tubing adheres to the choroid plexus in the ventricle and removal causes bleeding in the ventricle, a serious complication. We were fortunate tonight; all went well. I placed a new tubing in the ventricle with a new flush valve, connecting all to the tubing to the heart, with particular attention that it was well secured. She went to the recovery room by 4 a.m. and the following morning was much improved, and went home in two days.

Although the parents were told a great deal about shunts and malfunction, until this night, the hazards were theoretical, not real. Now the complications were real and her parents realized that they would worry for the rest of their lives. Bridget would always need access to acute neurosurgical care in case of occlusion of the shunt, a new reality. Not only might the shunt plug, it had the potential for being infected, each time revision occurred.

When I arrived in Peoria, children in the downstate, requiring a shunt, were treated in Chicago. I placed a number of those shunts at the Neuropsychiatric Institute in Chicago. I talked with the State of Illinois Division of Services for Crippled Children (DSCC) about caring for the children locally. DSCC regulations required board certification. Two years of clinical practice were necessary before I could sit the American Board of Neurological Surgery Examination. After a good deal of thought, the DSCC office permitted me to treat hydrocephalous patients under their care. Several years later, I was certified as described in an earlier chapter and continued to work with the DSCC to provide pediatric neurosurgical care. Passing the Board examination increased their level of comfort.

Hydrocephalous: Participating in the Evolution of Care

As I finished medical school in 1956, Dr. Donald Matson, the pediatric neurosurgeon at the Boston Children's Hospital published in the *New England Journal of Medicine* a paper entitled "Current Treatment of Infantile Hydrocephalous" describing his experience. At the time, Boston Children's and Children's Hospital of Philadelphia (CHOP) were leaders in children's care in the United States. Their best experience was with an operation that involved removing a kidney and threading a tube from the brain to the ureter allowing cerebrospinal fluid to drain through the urinary system. There were virtually no surgical deaths with this procedure, but constant loss of fluid and electrolytes contained in the cerebrospinal fluid created a chemical imbalance. A life-threatening meningitis infection developed in six to eight percent of the patients. The ventriculo-ureteral shunt was the best choice in 1956 but imperfect.

An interesting secondary effect of this work was the development of kidney transplantation, for which a plastic surgeon, Dr. Joseph Murray, received the Noble Prize in 1990. The procedure resulted in the availability of a healthy kidney. The availability of these kidneys stimulated the research of Murray and Francis Moore developing kidney transplantation at the Peter Bent Brigham Hospital in Boston.

In 1949, at the Children's Hospital of Philadelphia, Drs. Frank Nulsen and Eugene Spitz were working on a shunt with a valve to let the cerebrospinal fluid into the venous system in a one-way direction. In 1955 the son of John Holter, a machinist, was cared for at CHOP. Holter's son had hydrocephalus, and Holter was determined to develop a reliable, safe valve. The result was the first early valve, the Spitz-Holter valve utilizing silicon. The first valve was inserted in 1956. Large numbers of these valves were inserted, and Spitz never published the CHOP series. This shunt was a world-changing event in the care of hydrocephalous, allowing diversion of cerebrospinal fluid from the lateral ventricle to the internal jugular vein.

Late in 1956, Dr. Pudenz at the Huntington Hospital in Pasadena published the development of a shunt from the ventricle to the upper aspect of the right atrium of the heart via the jugular vein. His shunt employed a polyvinyl tubing initially, and he devised a slit valve that sat in the atrium of the heart. The first shunt was placed in a patient on April 4, 1955. He quickly changed to silastic and at the time of publication of the results, had operated on 23 patients. He demonstrated that the catheter should be in the right atrium of the heart, not in the jugular vein to function consistently. The tubing in the jugular vein tended to clot, causing shunt malfunction.

At the Illinois Neuropsychiatric Institute, we used the ureteral shunts with some success. In 1959, I placed a Pudenz shunt in a three-month-old baby, the first ventriculoatrial shunt placement performed at the NPI. We determined the proper location of the cardiac catheter with a portable chest x-ray. The tip of the catheter was to be at the level of the 6th thoracic vertebrae. Later we discovered that if we filled the cardiac catheter with saline and monitored with an EKG, we could determine the position of the catheter. When the P wave in the EKG became diphasic, the catheter was in the proper mid-atrial position, thus eliminating the need for an intraoperative x-ray.

The hydrocephalus problem was not solved; biological problems are never as simple as they appear. Over the next several years after my return to Peoria, several serious problems with the atrial catheter became apparent. If the system became infected, it sometimes resulted in infection of the tricuspid valve in the heart, often with valve rupture, heart failure and death. The catheter valve was sitting just above the tricuspid valve in the right side of the heart.

Some of the patients who had a shunt infection later proved to have decreased kidney function. Further study revealed some of the shunt patients were developing glomerulonephritis with impaired kidney function, sometimes progressing to irreversible end-stage renal disease. An immune response, often to Staphylococcus Epidermidis infection, resulted in the deposition of immune complexes in the kidney.

A new shunt that did not involve the circulating blood was needed. Fortunately, a new iteration permitted placement of the catheter in the abdomen, the cerebrospinal fluid flowing to the peritoneal space (the space containing the abdominal contents). The cerebrospinal fluid was absorbed there, avoiding heart and kidney damage. Dr. Tony Raimondi at the Cook County Hospital in Chicago published a paper in 1967 describing his successful placement of an abdominal catheter in 67 patients. I gradually converted to peritoneal shunts, although initially concerned they would not be reliable.

Parents still lived with constant worries regarding shunt malfunction, and less frequently, the threat of shunt system infection. The latter usually occurred at the time of a revision, so work continued to diminish that threat. Dr. Maurice Choux from Marseille, France brought what seemed an unbelievable report to the Cushing meeting; over 1000 shunt operations with infection occurring in well under 1% of the cases. He accomplished this by never touching the skin after the initial incision, not permitting entrance to the operating room after beginning the procedure, and not permitting anyone in the room unless essential for the operation. Choux eliminated all non-essential elements in the operating room, diminishing the risk of contamination. Our results steadily improved with the application of similar policies.

Over the years, a child free of shunt dependence remained

an elusive goal. Third ventriculostomy, an operation opening the third ventricle directly into the subarachnoid space around the brain bypassing obstructions, had been done for many years. Prohibitive complications produced by injury to critical surrounding brain structures limited its application. The technology available was just too inadequate to do the procedure well. We didn't see well enough, and the instruments were large. This operation permitted the cerebrospinal fluid to pass directly from the ventricles to the space around the brain for absorption, avoiding a shunt, no foreign body to become infected or obstructed. Endoscopes, initially developed for looking into sinuses and other applications, were applied to looking into the spaces in the brain. Now, this operation could be done with a tiny incision and much less risk as micro endoscopic instruments improved. This is a recurring theme in medicine; a sound theoretical concept only consistently accomplished when the appropriate technology permits safe, consistent execution.

Dr. Julian Lin, who came from the University of Texas in 1996 to train in neurosurgery at the University of Illinois, served a pediatric neurosurgery fellowship at The University of Tennessee and Saint Jude Hospital and returned to the Illinois Neurological Institute (INI). He developed a program using endoscopy to perform third ventriculostomy in selected patients; this treatment allows a fraction of the hydrocephalic children to be successfully treated without a shunt.

Significant progress has been made in the care of these children over the past fifty years, but many children remain dependent on the integrity of their shunt for life. Shunt revision remains a common procedure on all pediatric neurosurgery services, and parents of hydrocephalic children remain fearful of shunt malfunction.

Physicians' Evolving Approach to Blood Transfusion

Eric Able had just begun high school and was experiencing daily headaches. In early October, he started to vomit in the morning. Initially, his parents felt the problem was transition to high school, and their pediatrician agreed. However, he was progressively worse each day, and his walk became unsteady. When his pediatrician called late Friday afternoon, I arranged to see Eric urgently, Saturday morning. Examination revealed papilledema, swollen nerve heads in his eyes, indicating increased pressure in his brain. Eric's walk was unsteady, and he also had nystagmus, his eyes were jumping on lateral eye gaze.

I was confident Eric had a tumor in his cerebellum near the midline, since finger to nose testing was normal, suggesting the cerebellar hemispheres were not involved. I explained to Eric's parents he had a brain tumor, and there was reasonable hope in his age group it would prove to be the common benign brain tumor of childhood, a pilocytic cystic astrocytoma. Urgent surgery should be done before the papilledema caused permanent loss of vision. Eric's father wanted to proceed with surgery, then informed me they were Jehovah's Witnesses. I must accomplish the operation without transfusion of blood products. This decision was particularly challenging because Eric was a child, and his parents were making this critical decision. After a sleepless night, I concluded it was possible to do the operation without transfusion. If it proved to be the lesion I anticipated, a pilocytic cystic astrocytoma, blood loss would be small. If it were something else, I would stage the procedure. I discussed management of surgery with anesthesiology. They were adamant, and would not put the patient to sleep for surgery if the option to transfuse blood products was unavailable.

Eric's parents elected to urgently travel to a center in Detroit specializing in the care of Jehovah's Witnesses. I arranged a transfer without delay, and surgery was timely. Fortunately, the tumor was the hoped-for benign cystic astrocytoma. I saw Eric for his postoperative follow-up examination in three weeks; he recovered well without neurological impairment.

In the ensuing years, surgeons have become steadily more cautious concerning blood transfusion. At the time of Eric's surgery, virtually every patient on the neurosurgery service had a blood type and crossmatch, in preparation for transfusion. A crossmatch now is done only when thoughtful planning indicates a significant potential need for blood transfusion. In the '60s, a single unit transfusion was commonplace. It is now a reason for peer review. Blood loss in that range can either be reduced or managed without transfusion. Surgical technique and management of blood loss have improved. When significant blood loss is anticipated, cell saving units allow the return of the patient's blood to their circulation. Elective surgery sometimes utilizes the patient's banked blood in preparation for the planned surgical intervention, decreasing transfusion risk.

The rights of children are more adequately recognized, and there is legal recourse if a physician feels that a parent's decision is detrimental to the child's health. Today, I would operate on Eric with the support of our anesthesia service with more confidence than 1963. Blood and blood products are utilized more thoughtfully, after 50 years of additional experience. Another example of today's dogma is tomorrow's mistake.

Surgical Microscope Zurich

In the early '60s, surgical loupes for magnification and fiber optic headlights were improving. Lighted brain retractors were utilized in narrow, deep exposures. We just could not see delicate structures deep in the brain very well. A benign craniopharyngioma, adjacent to the pituitary gland, required delicate dissection of the distorted optic nerves and carotid arteries in the base of the brain. Inadequate visualization limited progress in complex surgery.

In the mid-'60s, a few papers appeared describing accomplishments in surgery utilizing the surgical microscope. The microscope provided magnification and intense lighting of the surgical work area. Dr. Leonard Malis at Mount Sinai and Dr. J. Lawrence Pool at the Neurological Institute of New York and Dr. Ted Kurze at University of Southern California (USC) in Los Angeles discussed their work with the microscope at national meetings. They used the Zeiss microscope utilized by ear surgeons for a decade. Dr. Gazi Yasargil, a young Turkish neurosurgeon, working in Zurich did microscopic research work on small vessel anastomosis, while visiting Dr. Peardon Donaghy at the University of Vermont. He returned to Dr. Hugo Krayenbuhl's department at the University of Zurich. A year after returning, he announced a course in microsurgery at the Kantonsspital Zurich. I decided to attend this first program in 1968, realizing that competence in microsurgery would rapidly become essential in cerebral vascular and brain tumor surgery.

This was the first of three twentieth-century revolutions in Neurosurgery: 1. Microsurgery, 2. Non-invasive imaging diagnosis with CT and MRI, and 3. Computer-guided surgery based on precise digital imaging.

I arranged to attend the course held November 14-21, 1968. I had never been away from the United States; this was an adventure. I flew Swiss Air from Chicago to Zurich. The strength and quality of the coffee served, and the cuisine on the flight was an introduction to Europe. I landed in Zurich, took the train to the Bahnhof and found my way to the small hotel in the old city within walking distance of the University hospital. The exchange rate was four SF to the dollar; thus my hotel was $7 per night with breakfast. A shoe shine was provided. Again wonderful strong coffee the next morning and my first croissant!

After a short walk to the University that morning, I met the small group attending the course, largely German and Scandinavian, with a few French and English neurosurgeons. Two young Americans, Dr. Joe Maroon from Indiana University, and Dr. Ed Seljeskog from the University of Minnesota, had just finished training and were sponsored by their departments.

We spent each day in didactic sessions, followed by hours of work on the microscope practicing small vessel anastomosis with 10-0 suture, the first time I had worked with anything that fine. Yasargil had modified many of the instruments, and each table had a full set. Although I had been operating eleven years, the concentration and precision involved were uniquely fatiguing, and I felt remarkably clumsy.

The first evening, a welcoming dinner was held at Kunsthalle Zurich. Professor Krayenbuhl welcomed everyone in French, German, and English. Fortunately, the universal language of the group was English. Generally, the group, especially the Swedes and Germans, were enthusiastic. The French neurosurgeons stayed in their section of the laboratory, perhaps a reflection of discomfort with English, the language of the course. Enthusiasm was not universal. An English aneurysm surgeon sitting in the back of me, Dr. Alan Richardson, was unimpressed and felt that the microscope was totally unnecessary!

One morning, I was able to leave the lab for a short time and watched Dr. Jean Siegfried perform several radiofrequency lesions in the basal ganglia for Parkinson's disease with exceptional skill. On each occasion, Dr. Siegfried did not make the radiofrequency lesion until Dr. Krayenbuhl approved, my introduction to the Germanic Geheimrat system, so unlike American democratic medicine.

Since they had just finished their residencies, and I had been in practice for seven years, I took Joe and Ed to dinner at the Kronenhalle Restaurant, at Ramistrasse 4, Zurich. The restaurant, founded in 1921, early on provided meals for many artists in exchange for their art. The owners, Gottlieb and Hulda Zumsteg, developed an extensive collection of works by Chagall, Matisse, Miro, Picasso, and Giacometti that hang on the walls of the restaurant. I had my first serving of entrecote with rosti. I was impressed by the delicious potato dish and the manner in which it was served. The waiter put a portion on the plate, then after that was consumed, served the remainder which had been covered with a metal dome to retain the warmth. A long way from Peoria!

At the end of the course, I walked down Bahnhofstrasse to do family shopping. I entered a six-story watch store and purchased a small Cellini Rolex for Gladys. I purchased some small Swiss toys for Katherine, Eric, and John. A long walk in the old town with dinner at Gleich, a unique old vegetarian restaurant finished the day. The return to Peoria was uneventful and anticlimactic for this new world traveler. The first neurosurgical revolution had started for me with this international excursion.

Craniopharyngioma: Zurich's Lessons Applied

Betsy Schwartz, a ten-year-old fifth grader at Whittier School in Peoria, was having trouble. She missed school because of a morning headache and vomiting for the past month, and she complained her poor vision was making her homework difficult. Her pediatrician asked me to see her two weeks after my return from Zurich. Betsy was a pleasant young girl who was a little overweight, and frightened by what was happening to her. She could not see in the periphery, on either side. When I checked her peripheral vision by wiggling fingers at the periphery, she had a bitemporal visual field deficit. This indicated a problem where the optic nerves join one another, at the base of the brain, the optic chiasm.

A skull x-ray revealed calcifications just above the sella turcia, the space for the pituitary gland, in the skull base. All of this suggested a diagnosis of craniopharyngioma. This benign brain tumor, common in children, caused difficulty with optic nerve function, hydrocephalous because of blockage of cerebrospinal fluid circulation, and changes in hormone function. The tumors, although not malignant, are difficult to cure because removal from the critical structures, at the base of the brain, risks damage to these structures. An operation would be my first utilization of the microscope, after Zurich.

I arranged to proceed with the operation using the Zeiss ear microscope at the Methodist Hospital. The only objective lens was 200 mm, providing less working distance than the 250 mm lens I used in Zurich. This made introduction of instruments into the operative field more difficult. I planned an all-day procedure, beginning early in the morning, the only operation that day.

I made a long incision in back of the hairline, brought the forehead scalp forward and created a large door in the skull, in the right side of the forehead. After gently lifting the frontal lobe of the brain, the large cyst of the craniopharyngioma tumor came into view. Opening and draining the cyst created room to work. I began to gently remove tumor from the carotid arteries and optic nerves, at the base of the skull, aided by the magnification and light provided by the microscope. The ability to separate the tumor from the arteries at the base of the brain, accurately, with sharp dissection, with bright clear vision, was absolutely thrilling. I had been performing brain tumor operations for ten years, and this was the first time the vision and the light made the work easy.

After extensive tumor removal, I had the upper basilar artery and the anterior aspect of the upper brainstem exposed. I was seeing these structures from the front, for the first time in my career, with magnification and remarkably bright light. Neurosurgery was transformed. The day had passed rapidly, and nine hours after starting, I placed the final suture in the scalp and helped lift Betsy off the OR table.

Betsy awakened promptly, and her vision was as good as before surgery. There was no apparent neurological damage. She did have diabetes insipidus, a condition related to change in the control of urinary concentration by the posterior pituitary gland and pituitary stalk. This caused production of excessive amounts of urine. I produced diabetes insipidus by surgical injury to the pituitary stalk despite the use of the microscope. This required careful treatment with vasopressin hormone injections, for the first week, then improved.

Betsy steadily recovered, and returned to the fifth grade with improved vision. She had a significant problem with weight gain, an almost universal experience in children with craniopharyngioma surgery related to changes in the diencephalic area of the brain.

In the next few years, neurosurgeons continued to debate the advisability of attempting complete removal of these tumors with the risk of injury to the diencephalon. Sadly, eight years later, Betsy had a recurrence of her tumor. I had left a small nest of cells that I did not see at the time of the original operation. We now do a more limited removal, if the risk of brain injury is apparent, and utilize highly focused Gamma Knife radiation to control the remaining cells that lie there, to avoid recreation of the tumor. Now, the goal is control of the tumor with a better quality of life than we were achieving with our attempts at complete removal.

Saint Francis Hospital committed to the purchase of a Zeiss OP 1 microscope with several objectives and a full set of Yasargil microsurgical instruments, in the next several months. Microsurgery had entered the Midwest. Interestingly, at the Interurban Neuro-surgery Meeting, held at the University Club in Chicago the following spring, the consensus of the participants at the meeting: "loupes and headlight are completely adequate, and the micro-scope adds little".

In a relatively short time, Saint Francis Hospital committed to, first in the Midwest, a Contraves microscope that Zeiss developed working with Yasargil and a rocket guidance company in Zurich. I was now able to move the microscope with a bite block between my teeth. The switch released the locks on the balanced micro-scope, allowing me to move the scope while operating with both hands.

The first of three significant revolutions in neurosurgery occurred in '60s. We could now see what we were doing in surgery; two more revolutions would occur in the next two decades; imaging allowing us to better see problems in the brain and spine before surgery, and image computer guidance bringing precision and decreased invasiveness to surgery.

Lumbar Disc Operation: Success then Disaster

Dr. Larry Fifield, a 49-year-old internist who practiced primarily at the Methodist Hospital, called and asked my advice. He had been playing singles tennis, ten days before, and after a particu-larly vigorous session, noted back pain and pain radiating into his right buttock. Over the next several days, the pain became intense, radiated into his calf, and he noted some numbness in his great toe. The morning of his call to me, his right foot begun to "slap" when he walked because he could not pick up the front of his foot and the pain in his leg was more intense.

I saw him in the office that morning with his lumbar spine x-rays. He could only bend forward about 10 degrees (normal 70-90 degrees), and he had pain on lifting his right leg at 10 degrees (normal 60-80 degrees). When I lifted his left leg, he had pain in the right leg, a crossed straight leg raising test indicating severe nerve root compression in the spine. He could not lift his right foot against resistance.

Clinically, he had a classic compression of the 5th lumbar nerve root caused by disc rupture between the 4th and 5th lumbar vertebrae. His spine x-rays were normal, he was in good health, and the remainder of his physical examination was normal. It was mid-April and Larry planned his annual canoe excursion into the Boundary Waters Wilderness area in July. He was anxious to continue practicing medicine, and wanted assurance he would be ready for the canoe trip in July.

In that era, I often did a lumbar hemilaminectomy for ruptured disc based on a clinical diagnosis, reserving myelography for patients lacking clear clinical localization. Later, virtually all patients had myelography, and often CT after myelography, before surgery. After the development of MRI, the diagnosis was made non-invasively. With Larry's clinical localization, I proceeded to surgery without myelography relying entirely on the history and physical examination.

The following morning, I did a lumbar hemilaminectomy, creating a small opening in the roof of the spinal canal and exposed the origin of the 5th lumbar nerve from the dural sac containing the spinal fluid and the nerves of the cauda equina. As expected, a large fragment of disc cartilage was distorting the nerve. This was carefully teased out, and the remainder of the degenerated disc removed, and the surgery finished. The operation took 80 minutes, and was uneventful. His leg pain was gone that evening, and unexpectedly, his weakness began to improve in the next several days.

In the '50s and early '60s, patients were kept at bed rest for several days after lumbar disc surgery and often were in hospital 6-7 days. Larry, being a motivated and confident physician ignored the rules, progressed rapidly, and went home on the fourth day.

Larry called me on the 8th day after surgery, saying he was having severe back pain and could not get out of bed. He lived three blocks from our house on Moss, so I made a house call, going up to his bedroom, on the second floor. He found it difficult to move in bed, his wound looked fine, and his leg function was normal. I felt he had discitis, an inflammatory process in the disc. Discitis was poorly understood in that era and was thought usually to not be bacterial in origin.

The symptoms usually lasted 8-12 weeks, resolving spontaneously with a bone fusion occurring at the disc level. An excellent long-term pain-free result after a prolonged period of excruciating back pain requiring immobilization was the expected course. The lab tech drew a blood sample for an erythrocyte sedimentation rate test, which was elevated to 100 compatible with my diagnosis of discitis. Purely on the basis of that clinical evaluation, I treated him with bed rest and anti-inflammatory medication. No canoe trip to the Quetico this year! I certainly was not a hero to him or to his canoeing partner, Dr. Joe Penny, an orthopedic surgeon.

Over the years, we have developed more understanding of this process. Although a sedimentation rate test is still used to follow the patient's course, the patients often have an MRI scan that is diagnostic of discitis. An image controlled needle aspiration of the interspace is done, for bacterial cultures. Some patients have an identified bacterial cause, and are treated with antibiotics, shortening the course of the process. Postoperative lumbar discitis remains a rare, painful, and expensive complication of disc surgery. Over the years, I have had 3 or 4 more patients with this problem. My first discitis, occurring in a physician friend was distressing and memorable. It is an important reminder that even in simple, usually successful surgery, problems can and do arise. Careful thought and discussion by the patient and surgeon before embarking on a surgical course is always important.

Intracranial Aneurysms:
A Long and Winding Road

In the late '50s and early '60s, the care of patients with subarachnoid hemorrhage (blood in the fluid surrounding the brain) caused by rupture of aneurysms and arteriovenous malformations was in its infancy. Early work was done in New York; London and Toronto, Ontario Canada; London UK; and Scandinavia. Chicago and the NPI were not leaders in this specialty. Subarachnoid hemorrhage caused by rupture of an aneurysm was not uniformly recognized, and if recognized, often was treated with bed rest in a quiet room until the patient was well, or died from repeat hemorrhage. Relatively few patients with subarachnoid hemorrhage were admitted to the University of Illinois Research and Educational Hospital(R&E). The R & E had a small emergency room, and these patients were not sent from outside hospitals. Therapeutic nihilism regarding subarachnoid hemorrhage existed in Chicago medicine.

In the neurosurgery department, Dr. Oscar Sugar was interested in subarachnoid hemorrhage, as part of his developing vascular program. Patients presenting with bleeding in the cerebrospinal fluid about the brain were treated with bed rest in a dark quiet room for 10-20 days, then had carotid angiography. A vertebral and basilar artery study was performed only if the carotid study did not reveal a cause for hemorrhage. At the NPI, Dr. Sugar and Dr. Holden pioneered percutaneous puncture of the vertebral artery for angiography in 1949. Necessary sophisticated, rapid film changing equipment was unavailable, thus vertebral angiography was rarely done. I had an interest in aneurysm management, but it was not a departmental priority.

Before embarking on the winding path of aneurysm care, my primary future career interest, I will review the state of the art, as it was in the late '50s. This involves troublesome technical detail, but illustrates the stepwise evolution of complex medical care with multiple worldwide contributors. While I was chief resident, Wylie McKissock, Kenneth Paine, and Lawrence Walsh reported 772 consecutive cases of ruptured intracranial aneurysm managed in London at St. George's Hospital, The National Hospital, and The Hospital for Sick Children in the July 1960 *Journal of Neurosurgery.* (1) These were the major London teaching hospitals providing neurosurgical care. Two hundred sixty six patients had a carotid ligation, and 151 had a "definitive craniotomy". A carotid ligation closed the carotid artery in the neck to decrease the pressure on the aneurysm in the brain, hopefully reducing the risk of repeated bleeding. A definitive craniotomy involved a brain operation clipping the neck of the aneurysm leaving the normal circulation unchanged. The mortality rate in the craniotomy group was 38 percent. They concluded that surgical treatment of ruptured intracranial aneurysm failed to lower the mortality, unless a large hematoma (blood clot) was present, and was removed. This paper did not encourage those seeking to improve the care of patients with brain bleeding with surgery. This publication summarized the state at one of the world's leading centers for neurosurgery. Indeed, not a field for the faint of heart.

Dr. J. Lawrence Pool at the Neurological Institute of New York was an American pioneer in the use of the microscope in operating upon aneurysms. He devised an operation that involved opening both sides of the front of the skull, elevating the brain, and placing temporary clips on the blood vessels leading to the aneurysm to prevent bursting of the aneurysm during the process of clipping. He progressively dissected the blood vessels and clipped the base of the aneurysm preserving the normal circulation. His was one of the early attempts at precision surgery in this complex problem. In the January 1961 *Journal of Neurosurgery,* Pool reported bifrontal craniotomy and routine use of temporary clips in anterior communicating aneurysms. His study included 28 patients; the mortality rate was 7 percent by utilizing hypothermia (cooling of the body) to 28C. (2) At that time, this was cutting-edge care in the United States and the most encouraging results reported to date. In 1963-65, by consistently adding hypothermia, he achieved remarkable results in treating intracranial aneurysms, significantly better than the English experience. Dr. Pool had applied the light and magnification of the microscope to create a precise operation.

Aneurysms arising from the basilar artery at the base of the brain were felt to be impossible to treat because of the depth of the exposure and the critical problem of circulation in the brain stem. Aneurysms of the basilar tip were essentially in the middle of the brain, considered a no-mans-land. Dr. Charles Drake in London, Ontario reported treatment of four patients in 1961 with two surviving the operation. He again published in 1965 with improving results in 14 patients. K.G. Jamieson from Brisbane, Australia, reported 19 cases in 1964, 7 patients treated for aneurysms of the basilar bifurcation. Ten of Jamieson's 19 patients died, and two were disabled. Both Drake's and Jamieson's papers were remarkably candid, reporting their surgical misfortunes in detail, providing a base for the progress of others. I did not take on this challenge until returning from Zurich in 1968. I sent several patients to Dr. Drake in the 1965-1970 period. With the availability of the microscope, I began using Drake's subtemporal approach. Later I utilized Yasargil's pterional technique and the "half and half" procedure described by Dr. Thor Sundt at the Mayo Clinic. After observing each of these surgeons in my travels, I brought the ideas and techniques home to Peoria. Watching Yasargil and Sundt was critical in this learning process. The impossible was gradually becoming possible.

Peoria was far from the centers with interest in aneurysm surgery. More patients with subarachnoid hemorrhage were arriving in the hospital, as physicians began to recognize the problem and referred them for treatment. Aneurysm care became my obsession. Initially, I did all of the angiography, but with the recruitment of Dr. Wright, his superb angiography provided better information needed for surgery. During this period, I had the opportunity to explore virtually every clip devised, angiographic techniques, as they developed, hypotension (lowering the blood pressure), hypothermia(lowering the body temperature to protect the brain), early and later surgery, and other permutations in management. 1961-1971 was a decade of rapid, exciting change.

In 1961, I treated some aneurysms of the carotid artery before its first major division (posterior communicating, ophthalmic, bifurcation) with carotid ligation in the neck with mixed results. With carotid ligation, we hoped to drop the pressure in the aneurysm avoiding further aneurysmal hemorrhage yet maintain enough blood flow to the brain to avoid a stroke. Reports from Duke University utilizing carotid ligation provided some support for this approach. A number of small connecting vessels at the base of the brain, called the Circle of Willis, form a variable connection between the major brain blood vessels. If the connections are fully developed, flow in the Circle provides adequate blood flow to the brain on the side of carotid occlusion. Unfortunately, the extent of the collateral connection is variable; some patients have a poorly developed Circle of Willis and have little protection against ischemia and stroke when the carotid artery is closed off.

To accomplish carotid ligation, I placed a box clamp around the carotid in the neck, under local anesthesia, with the patient awake. A stem came to the skin surface, allowing me to open or close the clamp, then after several days to remove the stem without opening the incision. At the NPI, we used a Salibi clamp, our modification of the Selverstone clamp. Initially, we closed it gradually over a two day period, opening if the patient began to have loss of function. Opening the clamp often drove a large clot that formed below the clamp, into the brain producing a massive stroke. A different approach was needed!

We next began to close the clamp immediately, only opening in the first minutes after closure if dysfunction occurred. This was better, but still unpredictable and did not provide adequate protection against rebleeding, hemiplegia, cerebral infarction (death of brain tissue secondary to loss of circulation), and death sometimes followed, yet some patients did well.

In the spring of 1962, I cared for a 45-year-old woman who was vigorously healthy before experiencing a subarachnoid hemorrhage from an internal carotid aneurysm. I applied a Salibi cervical carotid clamp under local anesthesia while she was awake. I opened the clamp four hours later, after the onset of mild left-sided weakness. Immediately, a complete left-sided paralysis developed that did not clear. It was an overwhelming experience to open the clamp causing the patient to become totally paralyzed, on the left side. The responsibility was absolutely clear and devastating. For months afterward, I reviewed in my mind the sequence of care in that patient. By late 1963, I had largely abandoned carotid ligation as a treatment for most aneurysms. I retained one Salibi clamp in my desk as a reminder of this journey and the damage I had done.

An intracranial operation with direct occlusion of the aneurysm, with preservation of all of the normal brain circulation, was the appropriate goal. Carotid or other proximal ligation of normal brain blood vessels was a poor compromise. I did a craniotomy on middle cerebral and anterior communicating aneurysms that were further from the base of the skull utilizing clips that were crude and imperfect. Initially, I used Cushing or Olivecrona silver clips, a clip that had a small wing on the back allowing removal, if the initial clip placement was unsatisfactory. Any attempted removal required pinching the wings to open the clip, a perilous step potentially causing rupture of the aneurysm or a tear in the parent artery.

We needed a clip that was readily applied, adjusted, and removed if necessary without tearing the artery and destroying the circulation of the brain. Dr. Schwartz in Saint Louis developed a clip with a large loop in the back that would allow removal, but the applier had a sizeable box-like holder, making it difficult to manipulate. The clumsy applier obscured the visualization of the anatomy. Dr. Mayfield working with George Kees in Cincinnati created a much smaller clip with a smaller applier that I used for several years while the hunt for the perfect clip and applier continued. Milton Heifetz in Los Angeles designed an even smaller clip and applier that I could utilize more safely. Drake in London, Ontario introduced the concept of an aperture at the base of the blades, allowing one to exclude an essential vessel from the closing blades of the clip and providing a higher closing pressure at the tip of the blades. Thor Sundt introduced a clip with graft material lining the clip, to be utilized as a salvage repair when the wall of a parent vessel was torn. This was termed a "clip graft". Neurosurgeons working with aneurysms were very creative. During this period, I tried many iterations of "the perfect clip" and visited and watched many neurosurgeons.

Later iterations by Dr. Yasargil in Zurich and Dr. Spetzler at Barrow Neurological Institute, provided clips with seemingly infinite variety, and low profile appliers easing application. At last, it was possible to see while the applier was going in, and the clips were readily removed, making aneurysm surgery more manageable and safer. Surgeons and engineers have utilized ingenuity and metallurgy to provide versatile titanium clips that are easily applied and removed and not deflected in MRI magnets up to 3 T.

In the 1960-70 period, I had problems with anterior communicating aneurysm patients awakening slowly with significant memory problems. Other neurosurgeons in centers worldwide were reporting a similar experience. The consensus was that we were damaging tiny branches (perforating vessels) that arose from the anterior communicating artery and the anterior cerebral artery that we were not able to see. We were producing small strokes in critically important areas of the brain. Dr. Lyle French in Minneapolis described removing the medial frontal lobe of the brain to achieve better exposure of the anterior communicating aneurysm, so I made a trip to visit him. I also visited Dr. Larry Pool in New York to watch his temporary clip technique with bifrontal craniotomy and did that operation as well. These collegial visits with neurosurgical experts were an important element in my technique development. Further improvement occurred after the Zurich trip in 1968 and the acquisition of a microscope. I finally was visualizing the small perforating vessels that I had been damaging leading to impaired postoperative function. The improved visualization of the small blood vessels significantly reduced the problems my patients were having with mental function after surgery for an aneurysm.

I lived in terror the aneurysm would rupture before I had defused it with a well-placed clip. The surgical field would fill with blood and surgery was no longer a meticulous, methodical dissection. I tried several preventive strategies. I first employed significant hypotension or lowering of the blood pressure, advocated by Dr. Drake in London, Ontario while dissecting the aneurysm with a mean arterial pressure at 60, softening the aneurysm. This reduced the blood supply to the brain, so the time available for the dissection was short, perhaps 5-10 minutes. Later, I used temporary clips on the vessel leading to the aneurysm. The brain was protected with barbiturates monitored with EEG burst suppression to confirm effective brain protection during the temporary vessel occlusion. Duke Samson at Texas Southwestern completed extensive research work delineating the time of safe occlusion. Lindsay Symon had begun this work in the laboratory at Queen Square, London. Again, these methods provided a short time window to get the job done.

Hypothermia to protect the brain was used intermittently, as knowledge was gained in its utilization in heart surgery. I first cooled patients to 28 C using a portable bathtub and ice cubes, when a prolonged period of temporary occlusion was anticipated. Gerald Silverberg at Stanford, working with the cardiac surgery service reported cases on cardiac bypass, done with profound hypothermia. He stopped the heart and circulation for twenty minutes to occlude the aneurysm. I visited him, and after working with our cardiac surgeons proceeded to employ full hypothermic arrest in a few extremely complex aneurysms.

This was a complicated process with a cardiac team and a brain team in the OR. Overall, I was not pleased with the result. A great deal of bleeding occurred when taking the patient off cardiac bypass. The patient required drugs while on cardiac bypass to prevent the blood from clotting (anticoagulants) and reversal was imperfect. As clips and dissection became better, the need for by-pass decreased and I did not pursue further development. The last patient that needed hypothermic cardiac bypass had a giant ophthalmic aneurysm, and would only tolerate 4 minutes of carotid occlusion. I could not control the aneurysm in such a limited time. I called Dr. Duke Samson in Dallas and arranged for a transfer of the patient to his department. I flew down to watch him perform the surgery. Surgery was difficult, but ultimately went well and the patient made a successful return to Peoria, in good health. This 25-year struggle illustrates the slow, halting progress in medicine with multiple contributors and no single hero. Each surgeon provided an incremental improvement.

Ruptured Basilar Tip Aneurysm, Application of Lessons Learned

Henry Lee, a 47-year-old, right-handed farmer, developed a sudden severe headache while walking to the field in the morning. He vomited, and returned home to lie down, felt even worse, and noted that his right eyelid was drooping. By noon, he went to the emergency room, in an adjacent small town. There, the physician did a spinal tap revealing blood in his spinal fluid. He called and I arranged for an ambulance transfer to Saint Francis Hospital. The ambulance arrived late in the evening. Dr. Wright performed angiography the next morning, revealing a 12 mm aneurysm at the end of the basilar artery pointing upward, backward, and slightly to the right.

A year had passed since my visit with Dr. Yasergil in Zurich. After a good deal of planning, arrangements were made for surgery the following morning with a plan to open the skull in the right temporal region in front of the ear and go under the temporal lobe as described by Dr. Drake. I administered intravenous urea while opening the skull. The urea produced a profound osmolar diuresis (a prodigious output of urine), resulting in the brain being very relaxed when I opened the brain covering. The brain was easily lifted from the floor of the skull, taking care not to injure the Vein of Labbe draining the blood from the temporal lobe.

With the microscope, I exposed the delicate arachnoid at the brain stem, opened it and gradually removed the available spinal fluid allowing me to raise the temporal lobe further and create a path to the tip of the basilar artery at the midline of the brain. I then saw the entire course of the third nerve and opened the fine arachnoid around this, allowing me to work above and below and gently move the third nerve, now visualizing the distal 10 mm of the basilar artery and the thin-walled aneurysm. The microscope allowed me to see the swirling blood in the aneurysm. There was a blood clot in back of the aneurysm, a clear indication that this was the leak site. I carefully removed some of the clot with suction and asked the anesthesiologist to drop the blood pressure to a mean arterial pressure of 60 mm. I dissected away several tiny perforating vessels on the back of the aneurysm, and I was able to introduce a Scoville clip, gently closing it without breaking the aneurysm. Earlier, I had used Mayfield clips that were larger and more clumsy, the smaller Scoville clip did not obscure my vision. The blood pressure was allowed to return to the previous level, and the clip remained closed. The subsequent wound closure was uneventful.

When I visited the recovery room, the patient was awakening and moving his arms and legs. His right pupil was dilated, the result of my manipulation of the third nerve, and the lid droop was now complete. He continued to awaken gradually, and the next day was alert with a headache and double vision, which cleared entirely in two weeks.

Mr. Lee, on the fourth day after surgery, told me that he was the father of eight children, noting that he did not wish to tell me before the operation, for fear it would make me anxious and tremulous while clipping his aneurysm. This had been the most anxiety filled aneurysm operation to date, but thankfully the hard work had been done by Drake and Jamieson. They had shown it could be done, and developed an early pathway, while working through their repeated failures. Their candid descriptions of encountered operative problems led the way.

Basilar tip aneurysms remain a challenge, but multiple anatomical avenues to approach them have been developed, depending on their configuration and their relation to the bony skull base. Yasargil and Sundt developed variations involving a pterional craniotomy and wide opening of the Sylvian fissure with later orbito-zygomatic arch approaches. Yasargil was the first to popularize an important basic concept; remove the skull rather than retract the brain, thus avoiding further brain injury. Others over the years expanded this work. Such a simple idea; take away the bone, rather than pull on the brain. Before Yasargil's insight none of us recognized the obvious. Safe removal of bone in the skull base became possible with the advent of high speed drills with diamond burrs permitting safe intracranial drilling. This concept was further extended with removal of orbital rim, allowing better visualization with less brain retraction. This is an example of the power of an individual's momentary creativity when the supportive technology becomes available. The final product so often is the result of multiple small additions to the knowledge base, rather than the work of a single brilliant individual.

Endovascular Therapy in Cerebrovascular Disease

For almost 50 years, aneurysms and arteriovenous malformations were approached from the outside through or under the brain, with clips and/or surgical removal. To approach them utilizing the existing vascular pathways, going up inside the blood vessels was an intuitively obvious, but difficult and slowly developing novel approach. Although some American neurosurgeons began to consider placing a balloon to occlude an aneurysm, Dr. Fedor Serbienko in Moscow created a balloon that could be placed then safely detached from the inserting catheter. His development of a detachment system was the critical step in the evolution of what was to become "endovascular surgery". Serbienko published his transformative work in the *Journal of Neurosurgery* in 1974. He had presented to the All Soviet Neurosurgical Congress in Moscow in 1971 but the world political state prevented early dissemination of this development beyond Russia.

My first response to Serbienko's paper was "I must go to Moscow and learn this technique" and went to the Peoria Public Library for a book to help me learn Russian. It soon became apparent I could not learn to speak Russian with a book. Russian seemed more difficult than German, and the Cyrillic alphabet was a mystery. Professor Gerard Debrun from Creteil, France visited Serbienko and, upon return to France, developed an active program to treat aneurysms with small balloons. The French remained at the forefront, in the early phases of endovascular neurosurgery, as the result of Debrun's timely visit.

Endovascular surgery developed rapidly. Dr. Kerber in California and neuroradiologists at both The University of California, San Francisco (UCSF) and The University of California, Los Angeles (UCLA), further developed silastic balloons to treat aneurysms. Instead of clipping the aneurysm from the outside, they were filling it from the inside utilizing the patient's existing pathways; aneurysms repaired without opening the skull.

The next dramatic change was the development of a thrombogenic coil by Dr. Guido Guglielmi, an Italian neurosurgeon working at UCLA with Dr. Fernando Vinuela. Guglielmi devised a method for detaching the coil from the introducing catheter with an electrolytic current. This unique invention allowed tiny coils to be placed in the aneurysm, packing it, and causing it to clot. The electrolytic current detachment allowed gentle removal of the catheter without disturbing the coil or the aneurysm. The aneurysm was treated non-invasively. The FDA awarded approval in September 1995.

The next step in the evolution of endovascular care was a neurosurgeon who does the full spectrum of treatments as appropriate, a neurosurgeon who was a microsurgeon and an endovascular surgeon. Dr. Nick Hopkins at Buffalo was a pioneer and a leader in this development, inducing neurosurgeons to actively participate in endovascular treatment. I made a trip to the University of California San Francisco (UCSF), to recruit someone with this training. I talked with Dr. Charlie Wilson, the chairman of neurosurgery, about who might be available. He recommended Dr. Stan Barnwell, an endovascular fellow who finished neurosurgery training with Dr. Wilson. Dr. Wilson asked my age and then told me "You need to plant an oak tree rather than an acorn" and encouraged me to pursue Stan. After several visits and thoughtful analysis, Stan elected to join the neurosurgery department at the University of Oregon. Recruitment to our fledgling department remained a challenge.

With further effort, we were able to recruit Dr. Ken Fraser from the University of Miami Jackson Memorial Hospital to develop an endovascular service at Saint Francis Medical Center. Ken had trained as an interventional neuroradiologist with Dr. Grant Hieshima on the pioneering service at UCSF. We began to use the detachable coil in 1995 as soon as they were available.

Over the ensuing twenty year period, our cerebrovascular team jointly evaluated each patient admitted with subarachnoid hemorrhage, and developed a treatment plan utilizing either an endovascular or a microsurgical solution. This multidisciplinary approach continues to evolve with approximately half of the aneurysms clipped and half coiled. I anticipate that the ratio will continue to gradually change with more patients receiving an endovascular treatment, as technological advances ensue.

We were providing excellent care, but not entirely prepared for the future. I continued recruitment for a neurosurgeon with endovascular training. Dr. Giuseppe Lanzino, who spent a year with Nick Hopkins, joined us after a fellowship with Dr. Spetzler at the Barrow Neurological Institute in 2000 to further develop endovascular surgery and assume responsibility for aneurysm microsurgery at the INI. I left aneurysm surgery with mixed feeling; aneurysms had been my primary interest for forty years, and I worked through each step in the development of the field. It was challenging and rewarding work, when all went well. A mistake in judgment or technique produced terrible disability for the patient; paralysis, speech loss, and mental changes. I redid those operations that did not go well time after time in my mind, often during the night, with a good deal of sadness. By 2002, I had clipped my last intracranial aneurysm and sleep was easier; Dr. Lanzino was in charge.

CT Brain Scans:
The Second Revolution, Imaging

Imaging of the brain was in a dramatic state of change in the early '70s. Gregory Hounsfield in England with EMI (Electric and Musical Industries, Ltd.) developed the computerized tomographic head scanner. EMI was a pioneer in recording and building gramophones, during WW II did radar work, and developed computer expertise after the war. Hounsfield developed the UK's first transistorized computer there in 1958, and subsequently developed the first CT scanner called the EMI Scanner. The company had an explosive success as the producer of the Beetles records in the '60s, and had the capital to develop this program.

When the first CT films were shown at the Cushing Society meeting, the English neurosurgeons working with Hounsfield showed images of a patient with a craniopharyngioma. I found it virtually incomprehensible that one could visualize a brain tumor without doing anything invasive; no spinal tap, no burr holes, no needles in the arteries, no injections. I, for a short time, questioned the validity and honesty of the process even considering fraud; a real skeptic. I finally accepted that a significant change was occurring in brain imaging. I began discussions with the Saint Francis

Hospital radiology department, and administrators Sister Canisa and Ed McGrath. They committed to the purchase of the first EMI head scanner in Illinois, and one of first US scanners, in 1973.

For the first time, we could visualize brain tumors, blood clots, and other problems without an invasive procedure on the patient! This scanner had a large water bag surrounding the head. Accurate placement in the water bag was critical, and it was a very prolonged process. The films did not provide fine detail and were pixilated, yet it was a disruptive advance in non-invasive diagnosis. Working a long day, we studied eight patients. For a short time, we were the only facility in the state with a scanner. Initially, only a neurologist, neurosurgeon, ophthalmologist, or otolaryngologist was permitted to order a CT scan because of limited capacity. This process was one of the first examples of an attempt at the rational utilization of limited resources. We performed few normal studies. Physicians excluded from the ordering process were quite angry, one of the early demonstrations of "rationing of care" in the United States.

It did take time and experience to realize what we were seeing, and have confidence in the result. A chronic subdural hematoma, a blood clot over the surface of the brain, proved to have a characteristic appearance, but the first several cases we confirmed with a cerebral angiogram because we had experience with that long utilized invasive study and did not have confidence in the new test. A demonstration of innate conservatism in medicine. Soon, we were seeing tumors and differentiating tumors by CT appearance.

There was a modest hiccup, in that competing manufacturers utilized different conventions for labeling the side of the images. Craniotomies were done on the wrong side from time to time around the United States until the problem was widely recognized. An early demonstration of the need for national criteria in medical care. CT scanning changed clinical neuroscience dramatically, and we were there at the onset. The risks and pain of intracranial air studies were eliminated and the long acquired skill sets associated with "air studies" were of no value. The microscope had provided the ability to see intra-operatively with precision, and this second development provided a non-invasive precise diagnosis; we could see significant detail. A blueprint available well before we operated provided better unhurried pre-operative planning. Hurried preoperative planning associated with air studies became history.

Several years later, the aperture in the machine was enlarged permitting the entire body to be scanned. The machines were faster and the images more precise. Scanning became so fast that patient throughput was determined by patient preparation time. Improvements in technology have permitted reduction of the radiation dose. Not all imaging problems have been solved, they have changed. Indiscriminate and excessive utilization remains a problem. With the burgeoning choices in imaging studies, an inappropriate choice is relatively common.

Childhood Pontine Hematoma

Sara Franklin, an 8-year-old girl, awakened with a severe headache after going to bed the previous night feeling well. Over several days, the problem persisted, and on the third day, she complained of double vision, was unsteady and began to vomit. The following morning, she had a definite weakness in the right arm and could no longer walk. Her speech was unaffected, suggesting the problem was in the brain stem rather than the left cerebral hemisphere. She was transferred to Saint Francis Hospital from another hospital eighty miles north of Peoria. Examination revealed a drowsy child who answered questions and complained of headache. She had double vision. She was unable to move her right eye outward indicating a right 6th nerve palsy. She had bilateral jerking movements of her eyes termed nystagmus. Her right arm and leg were weak; she could not lift them from the bed. With her speech and mental function intact, all signs pointed to a problem in the brain stem at the level of the pons.

The following morning, a CT scan revealed marked enlargement of the pons with characteristics suggesting an old liquefied blood clot. By late afternoon, her status had worsened. Although Walter Dandy, the neurosurgical leader at Johns Hopkins, after Dr. Harvey Cushing, had reported removal of a hematoma from the brain stem, few others had been reported, and I had never operated for this condition. Sara's condition was worsening rapidly; surgery was planned later that day. A catheter vertebral angiogram, done before surgery, demonstrated no evidence of an underlying collection of abnormal vessels, an arteriovenous malformation. In a relatively short time, imaging had so improved that it was possible to precisely localize the hemorrhage in the pons with the new CT scanner. Through an incision in back of the right ear, I removed some suboccipital bone, opened the dura, retracted the cerebellum, and exposed the side of the pons deep in the right cerebellopontine angle. The pons, just below the point of entry of the trigeminal nerve into the brain stem, was blue instead of the usual bright cream-white. With the Zeiss microscope, this was readily visualized and the point of entry into the brain stem selected. This was a point that could be opened without undue damage to brain stem function, a quarter inch incision was made, and the clot promptly drained with no further bleeding. The wound was closed, and the patient returned to the ward and seemed unchanged. By morning, she was much better and within 5 days was again walking and returned to her home in ten days. She was essentially normal within a month, and over the ensuing year seemed free of sequelae.

In the following nine months, I successfully operated upon two more similar, but older patients. I assembled pictures of the CT scans and began writing a paper describing this unique experience. Several weeks later, the *Journal of Neurology, Neurosurgery, and Psychiatry* arrived from England. It contained an excellent report of successful evacuation of a pontine hematoma, done at National Hospital Queen Square, and included a diagnostic CT scan. They had done a pneumoencephalogram, unnecessary in retrospect. CT scanning had made the diagnosis, and treatment of a formerly challenging lesion was relatively simple. The progress was already described in the literature; no need for an additional case report.

Progressive Blindness Stopped without Brain Surgery

Amy Adams, a 40-year-old mother of two teenaged children, had headaches, daily for two years. Three months before, she had an auto accident at an intersection which was deemed to be her fault. Amy did not see a car approaching from the left. She complained of fatigue over the previous six months, and stopped having menstrual periods. Progressive difficulty with reading and vision necessitated a visit to her optometrist's office, and he promptly called me.

Amy had loss of peripheral vision in the temporal fields of vision in both eyes and vision was 20/100 in the right eye and 20/200 in the left. Tests of pituitary function revealed a marked decrease in pituitary hormones. Carotid angiography revealed a massive pituitary tumor in the base of the brain.

Dr. John Henderson, shortly after returning to Peoria, visited the neurosurgical service at Case Western in Cleveland, where a friend was developing experience with the sublabial, transnasal, transsphenoidal approach to the pituitary gland. A small incision above the upper teeth, under the lip, provided a path through the nose to the pituitary. John had returned from Cleveland and accumulated the instrumentation required several months before Amy presented to us. In the past, I had treated these tumors by opening the right frontal skull, elevating the brain, and removing the tumor. Although generally successful, it was a major procedure with an extended postoperative period, and I often left some tumor in the sella turcia, the bony box in the skull base holding the pituitary.

Dr. Henderson felt he was ready, and I planned to assist. The morning of surgery, after anesthesia was begun, he packed the nose with gauze containing cocaine to decrease bleeding, then made a small incision under the upper lip, stripped the covering of the nasal septum, and gradually went through the nose to expose the sphenoid sinus with several fluoroscopic pictures to confirm our position. He found the enlarged sella enclosing the pituitary, chipped away the thinned bone, and opened the dura, the covering of the pituitary gland. The tumor was partially liquid and came out very easily with some fine scoop-like instruments. This was all done with the microscope permitting our manipulations to be easily seen despite the very narrow deep exposure achieved through the nose. We took a small piece of tissue from the hip area to close the base of the pituitary cavity, packed the nostrils with gauze containing an antibiotic, and put several sutures in the incision made under the lip. Amy awakened promptly in the recovery room, and was remarkably comfortable. Dr. Henderson left the packs in for four days, which was uncomfortable for Amy, and then removed them. Her vision improved by the day, and at a week, was 20/20 in both eyes and the temporal vision was improving. A new era in tumor surgery had arrived. In actuality, it was a reiteration of a rather old surgical procedure.

Transsphenoidal Surgery: Rebirth of an Old Procedure

When I arrived in Peoria in 1961, I felt most secure operating upon patients with pituitary tumors. Pituitary surgery was one of the most common operations during my chief year at the NPI. I made an incision in back of the hairline, peeled down the scalp of the forehead and opened a frontal craniotomy. The tumor was exposed with a lighted retractor and a headlight, utilizing loupe magnification. This technique was state-of-the-art in the United States and around the world, but significant change was imminent.

Dr. Jules Hardy, a French Canadian neurosurgeon from the Notre-Dame Hospital in Montreal, presented his experience with transsphenoidal surgery of pituitary tumors at the Harvey Cushing Society meeting in New York in April 1965. He had operated upon 20 pituitary tumor patients utilizing a trans-nasal operation with lateral fluoroscopic imaging for localization. His results were excellent, yielding recovery of vision with few complications. I was skeptical initially, feeling that he might be minimizing the difficulties and complexity of the operation, and awaited confirmation by others and further development of the technique.

This proved to be a truly disruptive development, and in the ensuing several years, Hardy returned with innovative work reporting selective removal of small tumors that were secreting hormones, with endocrine cure of the condition; a new world. Hardy began to use an ENT microscope in 1965 and soon realized that he could often identify and preserve the intact normal pituitary gland, a significant contribution to care of patients with pituitary tumor. Dr. Ivan Ciric was a fellow with Hardy, and returned to Chicago and did the first US modern transsphenoidal pituitary operation in 1967. Dr. Charles Wilson visited Guiot in Paris, at about the same time, and performed the first transsphenoidal surgery for acromegaly (pituitary gigantism) at the University of California, San Francisco in 1970.

After Dr. Henderson returned from Chicago in 1971, we arranged that he would go to Cleveland to learn the technique and we were soon treating most pituitary tumors in this fashion.

As has so often happened in medicine, this dramatic development was an application of an old technique, considerably changed by the availability of new technology, in this case, the surgical microscope and the radiology image intensifier. The microscope made it possible to see the surgery site precisely, and the image intensifier allowed one to monitor the relationship of operative activity to the brain above.

Dr. Cushing did his first transsphenoidal pituitary operation at the Johns Hopkins Hospital in 1909. In 1910, a Viennese otorhinolaryngologist, Dr. Oskar Hirsch, originated an endonasal transseptal operation. In the same period, Dr. Knavel in Chicago performed a transnasal approach. Cushing did this operation in Boston until 1929-1932, when he adapted the frontal transcranial approach. Dr. Norman Dott, a Scots neurosurgeon, worked with Cushing in 1924, and took the transnasal operation home to Edinburgh. Dr. Gerard Guiot, a French neurosurgeon in Paris visited Dott in 1956, was impressed by the transnasal operation, and performed it in Paris, adding fluoroscopic image intensification to increase safety. Jules Hardy trained with Guiot at Foch Hospital in Paris, and upon return to Montreal in 1962, applied the microscope to the operation. A circuitous process, Cushing-Dott-Guiot-Hardy resulted in a gradual worldwide reapplication of a transsphenoidal approach to pituitary tumor utilizing modern technology.

I was trained by Eric Oldberg, who was a resident with Cushing in 1928-1930 and hence, learned to resect pituitary tumors through

145

a right transfrontal craniotomy rather than transnasally, as Norman Dott had learned just several years earlier. The availability of the surgical microscope and image intensifier made a previously technically challenging operation readily accomplished, and changed the management paradigm for a pituitary tumor. Many pituitary tumors could be managed without opening the skull, and with significantly less morbidity. An old, imperfect operation significantly improved by technology, a story often told.

Epidural Hematoma

The call came Thanksgiving morning from Graham Hospital, 35 miles away. A five-year-old boy, Sam Pickens, had fallen from his bicycle, struck his head, was momentarily unresponsive, then awakened crying and was brought to the emergency room by his father. A skull X-ray failed to reveal a fracture. The physician in the emergency room asked that he be transferred because he had been momentarily unconscious. He arrived several hours later, awake and vomiting. The nurse called, indicating the child was alert, and I said I would come by on morning rounds.

I came to the pediatric unit at 10 a.m. Thanksgiving morning, and found the child unresponsive and not moving his left arm and leg. The nurse indicated the change had happened in the past ten minutes. His right pupil was large, and looking in his ear, his right eardrum was blue, showing that he had bleeding in the middle ear, usually associated with a temporal bone skull fracture. The child had all of the signs of the most serious neurosurgery emergency of childhood, an epidural hematoma, a blood clot between the skull and the dura mater, the tough outer covering of the brain.

I asked the nurse to call OR and tell them to get ready, as I lifted him in my arms and started to the operating room. We quickly clipped the hair about the right ear as the anesthesiologist was inserting an endotracheal tube in his windpipe, prepared the skin, and made a vertical incision in front of his right ear, exposing a temporal bone fracture. The skull immediately in front of the ear is so thin in a child that a fracture sometimes is not seen on x-ray. I rapidly opened the skull and a dark red clot extruded. The middle meningeal artery in the covering of the brain was torn with the fracture and resumed bleeding vigorously with clot removal. I coagulated the middle meningeal artery with the cautery and the bleeding stopped. The remainder of the clot was removed, the wound sutured, and Sam was taken to the recovery room. His right pupil was now small, and within an hour, he awakened. The Pickens family celebrated Thanksgiving three days later with Sam at the table.

An epidural hematoma in a child can be the most gratifying experience in the career of a neurosurgeon or the most devastating failure depending on as little time as 20 minutes. Too late and secondary damage in the brain stem means the child never awakens or has permanent neurological devastation. I later cared for a ten-year-old boy that was struck with a rock, admitted to a distant hospital and transferred after going into coma. Although I operated as soon as he arrived in our hospital by helicopter, both pupils remained dilated, he never regained consciousness and died. This child demonstrated the need for a system of care in rural areas serving patients injured at some distance from complex medical facilities.

The key to successful treatment of childhood epidural hematoma is the understanding of the involvement of the middle meningeal artery with the thin temporal bone and adequate suspicion of a temporal fracture when a child has bloody drainage from their ear, or their eardrum is blue. These are signs that the child must be in a facility that can immediately treat an epidural hematoma if it develops. My direct response to this was to redouble my efforts in teaching medical students and emergency room physicians to look at the eardrums of children after falls. CT scans now provide excellent images allowing accurate prediction of the risk of epidural hematoma. Prompt helicopter transfer occurs after CT scan identification of the problem.

Chapter 5

Medical Education, A Second Career Beckons 1970-1979

Education is not about filling a pail; it is about lighting a fire.

— W.B. Yeats

A Medical School: New Directions

In the '60s, a strategic decision to increase national medical manpower was made and a number of new medical schools were established in the United States. (1) Most were to be "community-based" medical schools utilizing existing non-teaching hospitals and medical staff. The objective was to increase the number of doctors providing primary care, without the cost of developing new research-oriented academic medical centers.

After much internal debate, the University of Illinois decided to enlarge the College of Medicine functioning at four sites, Chicago, Urbana, Peoria, and Rockford. Students enrolled the first year at Chicago or Urbana. The Urbana students, after the first year, would either continue in Urbana or move to Peoria, or Rockford, as M2 students. Since the University of Illinois had a large group of scientists on the Urbana campus, this seemed an efficient expansion, without excessive cost for additional basic science faculty.

The Peoria School of Medicine was established in 1970 with the appointment of Nicholas Cotsonas M.D. as the first dean. Temporary offices were established in downtown Peoria in the First National Bank Building. Initially, there were no conventional specialty departments, the faculty was organized in "disciplines". Virtually all faculty members were voluntary and each discipline was headed by a "coordinator" rather than a classic department chairman.

Classes for the initial student group transferred from the Chicago campus were conducted in the two downtown hospitals. With the arrival of the first full class, space was leased in a Bradley University building until the construction of a medical school building was completed. The University leadership wished to place the building away from all of the hospitals near Parkview cemetery (disparagingly referred to, locally, as the "Grove's Graves" site). Dr. Grove was Dean of the College of Medicine. The University developed the medical school at Rockford at a distance from the three existing hospitals, but the medical community did not wish that in Peoria. There was a fundamental disagreement regarding the role of the hospital in healthcare, which continues to the present. Dean Grove felt that outpatient care was critical to the function of the new medical school, and care within a hospital should receive much less emphasis. The Peoria medical community remained hospital-centric.

Mayor Carver was a major factor in obtaining federal urban renewal funds to permit building on a site adjacent to the two major teaching hospitals, forming a formidable downtown medical center. After great civic effort, the land was obtained and the medical school building was constructed just west of the Methodist campus opening in November 1976. We were on the way to a more conventional academic health care center.

I met Dr. Cotsonas in his Bank Building office and told him I would like a neuroscience department, incorporating all of neurology, neurosurgery, and basic neurological science. This was not the conventional arrangement in American medical schools. Dr. Norman Dott, a British neurosurgeon in Edinburgh, Scotland described his experience with such a structure to the Congress of Neurological Surgeons several years before. His lecture influenced my thinking regarding the organization of neurological care and education. Dr. Cotsonas intended neurosurgery to be in the surgery discipline, and neurology to be in the medicine discipline. After heated discussion, Cotsonas exclaimed, "this is not the Peoria School of Brain Surgery" ending the meeting. The important decision to create a clinical neuroscience program was ultimately made and neuroscience became a department in 1974. Dr. Cotsonas did not allow me to include basic neuroscience in the department, a disappointing compromise of my initial vision.

A prolonged search to fill the headship ensued. Although this was an unconventional department without residencies in neurology and neurosurgery, a number of candidates expressed interest in the position. The process was a period of interesting self-discovery. I wanted an innovative, superb department of neuroscience, and at the same time, was personally interested in developing and leading such a program. On critical self-analysis, I clearly lacked the experience and training for the role, but assumed with *hubris* that I would "grow into the role". I became Professor and Head in 1977, and spent the next twenty-seven years "growing". My partners and I formed the Neurological Associates, a multidisciplinary private practice, in 1968, intending to build a neurology and neurosurgery faculty and now it was time to execute the plan.

I chaired the initial curriculum committee as the faculty developed an "organ system" approach to the second pathophysiology year. Dr. William Albers, who led pediatrics, attended Case Western in Cleveland and experienced the value of the organ system curriculum structure. He provided support and guidance as we worked through the creation of the second year curriculum. While developing this program, we admitted our first class of 18 juniors and 3 seniors in September 1971 in transfer from the Chicago campus. The first M2 class of twenty-five students arrived in 1972, utilizing rented space on the Bradley campus for the didactic experience. This first full class entering as M2's graduated in 1975.

In the first several years, a faculty was assembled and we explored the requirements of teaching undergraduate medical students in multiple disciplines. Washington University in Saint Louis utilized the organ system curriculum and seemed a possible model. Although their mission as a private national medical school was quite different from our role as a public medical school serving the people of Illinois, their leadership helped a great deal. A visit to the new school at the Mayo Clinic provided insight into creating a program for a small medical school class, in a clinically oriented environment. Their challenges were similar to ours in Peoria, but they had more resources and a large faculty.

The immediate challenge was to create a good clinical experience for the transfer students from Chicago. A set of 20 cases illustrating important neurological problems provided a framework for the clinical neuroscience clerkship. We worked with groups of 3 to 4 students several days per week when they were on the clerkship, evaluating patients and reviewing the selected teaching case material. It was an exciting time; the students volunteered for this experience at Peoria. All of the faculty, although totally inexperienced in pedagogy, were thrilled with an opportunity to teach medicine. The excitement lasted perhaps five years, a long honeymoon.

The first full class consisted of 25 students who spent their first year in Urbana, opting for a somewhat "self-taught" independent learning experience. Most of the class were highly motivated and passed the National Board Part I examination after the first year, before arriving on the Peoria campus for the second year. Students usually took Part 1 of the National Board examination at the end of the second year. Student and faculty enthusiasm was boundless and infectious.

A 6 week neuroscience pathophysiology and pharmacology program was assembled in the 2nd year and a 4 week neurology and neurosurgery clerkship followed for 3rd and 4th year medical students. The next several years, I met with groups of 4 juniors every Wednesday and Friday afternoon, for two hours. The students presented 2 cases for analysis and review. They had the option of presenting any patient of interest, making the experience unpredictable and challenging; I never knew what to expect.

I learned a great deal about undergraduate medical education and participated in University committees to change the classic four-year curriculum to one that offered early exposure to clinical

153

medicine and basic science related to clinical problems. The classes were small, and most of the faculty were enthusiastic about this new opportunity in their lives. They were willing to work hard in this new venture. The new faculty members had difficulty understanding the student's knowledge base, and at times taught as if they were teaching third-year graduate residents instead of third-year medical students. We were in a fast-track learning mode. In less than two years, we had an accreditation site visit, my first such experience. I made the mistake of attempting to educate the site visitors regarding new curriculum design, the right way to conduct a medical education! That was not well received, and Dr. Cotsonas recommended a more humble approach.

During this first decade, a number of students pursued careers in neurosurgery, neurology, and neuroradiology. Mentoring them, while they explored graduate training, was rewarding. Dr. Richard Lister, a member of the first class, was our first student to enter a neurosurgery career. On completion of his residency at the University of Florida, he joined our faculty in 1980.

We were charged with developing continuing education for practicing physicians to improve the quality of medical practice in the downstate. The first official Continuing Medical Education (CME) program of the College of Medicine was given by the Neuroscience Discipline. "What to do When the Stroke Comes" was provided to 100 downstate physicians in an all-day session in the 7th-floor auditorium at Saint Francis Hospital in 1971. In reviewing the curriculum, the care we were discussing was state-of-the-art, but woefully inadequate by current standards. Our department subsequently provided an annual day-long neuroscience conference, over the years making some contribution to the quality of neurological care in the downstate.

The Faculty Assumes Their Role

A new medical school and an increasingly large residency graduate program were grafted on a private practice community with three hospitals staffed by "voluntary faculty". The teaching model differed from classical academic medical centers; it involved private practice physicians bringing their patients to the hospital. These physicians had a staff appointment in the hospital, and volunteered time for committee work and support work in the hospital. A few received modest part-time pay, if they devoted significant time to hospital administrative tasks. Virtually all of the faculty were donating as much as 4-6 hours per week, attracted by the novelty of something different.

Designation did not immediately create a functional faculty. Most physicians were away from the reality of medical school or residency for 10-20 years. Although well-meaning, enthusiastic, and expert in delivering clinical care, most had significant deficiencies as faculty. The students were arriving from Urbana soon. The faculty were unaware of what the students knew, nor did they know what the students needed to learn in the second year, an immediate challenge.

The second and third-year curriculum was developed by the committee on instruction, with support from educators on the Chicago campus. Programs were developed to assist faculty in the acquisition of teaching skills. Fortunately, the University of Illinois College Of Medicine was a pioneer in techniques of medical education, led by George Miller, and had staff with expertise in teaching physicians to be teachers. Getting the job done without these people would have been difficult. Although the University organization was by "discipline" without the usual formal departments, there was a helpful, strong departmental structure in Saint Francis and Methodist hospitals.

We lacked identification as faculty. After the first year, the faculty wore a clinical coat while on the clinical units and in conferences. There was some sensitivity about a "white coat syndrome" and finally, a striped blue faculty coat was selected. Pediatrics wore a brown coat, and the neuroscience faculty used a blue coat, and after a bit of electioneering, a faculty vote committed to the blue coat. Jack Henderson and his wife designed a U of I Logo for the shoulder, and we had a faculty identity that held up through the years. In recent years informality increased, scrub suits are worn on the units, and it is more difficult to identify faculty and residents.

Over time, the voluntary faculty model became unsustainable. The class grew from 25 to 55, and more residents enrolled, thus increasing teaching responsibilities. Gradually full or part-time faculty were employed, either by the University or the hospital. We were losing some of the excitement and looked somewhat more like a conventional academic center, yet lacked research structure.

After 45 years, we still are working on the optimum hospital and College of Medicine relationship. The hospital and the clinics are the "workshop" of the College of Medicine, yet there is incomplete transparency between the partners, with a resultant loss to the clinical, educational, and research enterprise. The committee structure of hospital and College of Medicine is not integrated. The health care system and College of Medicine computer systems lack functional integration. We undoubtedly share this problem with most academic centers in the United States.

Progressive Blindness: Vision Saved

Gerald McShane, third-year medical student, a member of the first non-transfer class at the University of Illinois College of Medicine at Peoria (Class of 1975), called at 7 p.m., to report he just finished examining Bill Phillips. Bill was a 19-year-old male student transferred to my service from another hospital, early that evening, with rapidly decreasing vision in both eyes. Gerry indicated that the patient had signs of increased pressure in his brain, when looking into his eyes. The nerve heads were swollen with hemorrhages in the retina (papilledema), and the patient had bruits (a whooshing sound) over his neck and entire head.

I went to the hospital that night and examined the patient with Gerry. We found profound papilledema in both eyes and bruits over both carotid arteries in the neck and across the back of the head. His visual acuity was reduced to 20/100 in each eye. I suspected an abnormal connection between the arteries and veins in the covering of the brain (dural arteriovenous fistula) causing a rapid increase in the pressure in the veins of the brain, impairing drainage of blood from the brain. The brain, located within the rigid skull, has a unique problem, a limited non-expandable space. If the blood cannot leave the brain promptly, increased pressure immediately develops. In 1974, dural arteriovenous fistulae were not studied extensively, and few clinical reports existed to guide us. I talked with Dr. Wright that evening, and he scheduled angiography for the next morning.

Angiography revealed the suspected dural arteriovenous fistula involving the main venous drainage of the brain in the back of the head. The posterior sagittal sinus, in the midline of the brain, and each transverse sinus passing near the mastoid were involved by abnormal blood vessel connections. This reduced the outflow of blood from the brain causing pressure evident in the optic nerve in the back of the eye.

Dr. Wright and I needed a treatment plan. There were few reports of successful management of a fistula this complex. Houser published a report from the Mayo Clinic in October 1972 describing 28 patients seen at Mayo from 1958, 11 with somewhat similar lesions. They had attempted direct closure in 3 of those patients. (1) Aminoff reported 16 patients from the National Hospital,

Queen Square, London. (2) One patient had muscle embolization of feeding arteries, and five had surgery. Neither paper provided surgical detail. We needed to reduce the blood flow a great deal before I could safely open the skull over this abnormality producing high blood flow immediately under the skull. The review of the literature did not provide a comprehensive treatment plan supported by clinical data. Dr. Wright planned to place a catheter in the arteries feeding the abnormal connections, and embolize them with small bits of muscle that I would take from the patient's hip area. Several sessions would be required to reduce the shunting and the blood flow to allow safe surgical treatment. The evening after the first embolization session, the patient had a great deal of headache in his neck and the back of his head, but remained alert and his vision was no worse. Two days later, Dr. Wright closed off a number of additional vessels, with a resulting similar reaction.

Several days after the embolization, I opened the skull over the involved areas and disconnected the venous pathway from the arteries in a procedure lasting almost eight hours. Bill awakened promptly from the operation without any brain dysfunction but with a severe headache that gradually improved over the next few days. In the ensuing week, the optic nerve swelling decreased and vision improved, and he returned home. An office visit several weeks later revealed that vision had returned to normal and no optic nerve swelling remained. Bill remained well as he started college.

Dr. Thor Sundt at the Mayo Clinic published a series of 27 patients nine years later, in 1983, providing his experience with this problem. This included a patient who died in surgery with uncontrolled bleeding, after elevating the bone flap. (3) Although the members of our department had an interest in this process, and subsequently saw many patients that were thoroughly studied by Dr. Wright, we did not publish our experience. This was an important omission because progress in care of rare conditions is made in small, incremental steps based on collective reported global experience.

In more recent years, with an improved understanding of the physiology and technology, most dural arteriovenous fistulas are treated entirely with endovascular catheter techniques involving a needle puncture in the groin and introduction of a catheter that is threaded to the fistula. The lesion is then closed off with embolic agents or clot inducing coils. Since 2000, I have utilized the Gamma Knife to treat some that are not readily treated with surgery or endovascular catheter techniques. The Gamma Knife causes the abnormal blood vessels to thicken and gradually close. Accumulated knowledge and experience over forty years allows less invasive treatment for most patients harboring dural arteriovenous fistulae, although some patients still require definitive surgery.

Academic Department Head, a New Career

Although a clinical neuroscience department was in place in 1974, a permanent department head was not appointed until 1977. A lengthy search surfaced a number of neurologists and neurosurgeons interested in exploring the position. Virtually all had reservations about the unconventional academic structure. Was this position in Peoria a wise choice in an academic career?

Dean Cotsonas was reluctant to consider me because of my sparse publication record, inexperience with graduate education, and impatient temperament. He resolved the issue by holding an election of the executive committee, allowing him to"share the blame" in the appointment. I was now a freshly minted "Professor and Head". The University did not provide an orientation to this new role. In that era, department heads in academic centers were selected for their scientific prowess, and the position required leadership skills not tested in the prior research and clinical career. Solving the leadership problem was clearly in my inadequate hands.

After five years as Head, in 1982, a formal Headship review was dictated by University statute. A review committee included faculty from other campuses of the University of Illinois College of Medicine and other Colleges within the University. Dr. Robert Grossman, the Professor and Chairman of Neurosurgery at Baylor College of Medicine in Houston was selected as the external visitor. Dr. Grossman had been Chairman at University of Texas Medical Branch before moving to Baylor. He was an experienced academician who reviewed the department carefully and gave me useful advice regarding further department development. The committee met with me and submitted a formal review of my performance. They felt I had accomplished a great deal in the five year period, but pointed out that I was autocratic, tended to concentrate on what had not been accomplished, and did not celebrate the success of others. A department head who urgently needed "fine tuning".

Their analysis was remarkably accurate, and difficult to accept. The struggle to improve my deficiencies continues to this day. At eighty-six, celebrating the success of others is easier, and I am content not achieving rapid culture change. Some lessons learned too slowly! The opportunities lost as a result of such foolishness still haunt me. The lesson learned: all administrators benefit from a firm coach that is brutally honest about their deficiencies and failures. Coaches are hard to find, and Presidents, Deans, and CEO's should insist that their major reports have a compatible coach.

The department in a medical school or a hospital is the most appropriate unit to achieve change. It is small enough and cohesive enough to deal with culture change, and problems, and to develop a long term strategy that can be executed. In looking at departments that have been successful in clinical care, education, and research, a key element is the department head. His/her ability to mentor each faculty member to their full potential builds academic careers. Combining individual faculty into a whole that is much greater than the sum of the parts is critical to the life of a department.

The headship is not an honorific, but a responsibility and a task that requires hard work, creativity, collegiality, vision, and drive. Some effective department heads sacrifice some of their own clinical and research interests to the greater task and responsibility that they have accepted. Department heads that continue primarily with their own clinical work or research often fail to achieve the potential of their department to the detriment of their faculty and students. Those that devote themselves entirely to administrative matters lose touch with clinical medicine; a balance is difficult. New department heads often do not understand the new responsibility as they enter the process. Universities continue to do a mediocre job in guiding their new department heads.

Stroke: The End of Therapeutic Nihilism

"What to do When the Stroke Comes" was the first full day continuing education program sponsored by the College of Medicine. The 7th-floor auditorium at Saint Francis Hospital was filled with practicing physicians, as we embarked on improving medical care in the downstate in 1971. We were developing treatments for aneurysmal subarachnoid hemorrhage and significant atherosclerotic narrowing of the carotid artery, the major artery leading to the brain in the neck. We offered little to patients who had an occluded blood vessel within the brain, either because of a clot, originating from the heart, or a clot developing in a branch vessel in the brain. Various protective agents were tried in large clinical trials with no apparent benefit. Dr. Garwacki did participate in multiple brain protective trials, while training in Detroit.

We were offering something, but not a complete menu "when the stroke comes".

Dr. Thomas Brott developed the first stroke network in the United States, in Cincinnati and Northern Kentucky, offering a system of stroke care serving a number of metropolitan hospitals and participating in early stroke treatment trials. I invited him as a visiting professor to update us on the work they were doing. These trends were discussed with hospital leadership and they agreed to support recruitment of a stroke neurologist to develop a rural stroke network. Watching stroke patients steadily worsen continued to be a "black cloud".

Dr. Cathy Helgason trained with Dr. Louis Kaplan, a pioneer in stroke neurology at Michael Reese Hospital in Chicago. She was a young faculty member at the Veterans Administration Hospital at the University of Illinois in Chicago. Cathy joined our department in 1989 to develop a stroke program centered at Saint Francis Medical Center. Progress and interest in stroke care began to build in the medical staff and the referring hospitals.

Cathy returned to Chicago after 18 months. The distance from Chicago and family support proved to be a much greater burden than Cathy or I anticipated. I failed to recognize the stressful change involved in her move from an established center in Chicago to a developing program outside of a metropolitan area. My search for a stroke neurologist began anew.

Dr. David Wang joined the neurology department in 1994, after completing a neurology residency at Henry Ford Hospital in Detroit and a stroke fellowship at Creighton University and Medical College of Ohio with Dr. Clark Milliken. He teamed with Jean Rose, RN, MS, manager of the neurological ICU. Over the ensuing several years, formal relationships were developed with surrounding rural hospitals. Thus, the largest rural stroke network in the United States evolved, encompassing 24 hospitals. Dr. Wang established a vascular neurology fellowship in 2005, and offered training to one fellow, each year.

A report in the *New England Journal of Medicine* (NEJM) galvanized the medical profession in 1995.(1)Tissue plasmino-gen activator (tPA), administered within three hours of symptom onset, improved the outcome in ischemic stroke. Something could be done for stroke. TPA soon acquired the popular name "Clot Buster". The stroke network now had a clear purpose. An available treatment created increased public awareness of stroke. This generated a change to activism in the neurology world. "Watch and wait" was no longer tenable in stroke. The era of neurology as a contemplative specialty was over. A CT scan was done to exclude hemorrhage, and treatment started as soon as possible. The "door to needle" time was the new metric measured, and reported. Neurological call coverage became important. Dramatic change was in the air!

Twenty years after the formation of trauma centers, a Primary Stroke Center accreditation was developed by the Joint Commission. The Stroke Center at OSF Saint Francis Medical Center was the first accredited in Illinois in 2000, the product of relentless drive by Dr. Wang and Jean Rose. A Comprehensive Center accreditation including competencies in neurosurgery, endovascular surgery, and rehabilitation was later developed. In 2012, the Illinois Neurological Institute at OSF Saint Francis Medical Center was the second to be accredited in the US as a Comprehensive Stroke Center. In 2015, the center admitted the largest number of stroke patients in the state, and is the site of many clinical research studies. Much had been accomplished since 1971. The 1995 thrombolysis paper was the game changer with intravenous thrombolysis in the first three hours, a standard of care making stroke management infrastructure important.

After intravenous treatment was established, the next question begging resolution remained: will directly taking the clot out of the artery give even better results? After multiple studies, confounded by rapidly changing technology, the question of the efficacy of intra-arterial intervention was resolved. Early studies did not indicate value because of technological limitations. In the first three months of 2015, 4 studies proved the value of intra-arterial intervention. These studies demonstrating the efficacy of endovascular clot extraction confirmed the importance of commitment to a comprehensive center. These developments are explored further in Chapter 8's consideration of cerebrovascular illness.

"I Want to be a Brain Surgeon" — First Residency Candidate

The first class of twenty-five students began making career choices while pursuing third-year clinical clerkships. Most students contemplated family practice, internal medicine, or pediatrics. They had chosen to attend this rural medical school committed to educating primary care physicians. But, as Robert Burns said, "The best laid schemes o'mice an' men gang aft agley", some students chose specialized, non-primary care specialties. This choice occurred more often in Peoria than Rockford. Large hospitals with specialty services and residencies provided role models for sub-specialty careers in Peoria.

Richard Lister was born and raised in Shipman, a small town in southern Illinois. Dick entered the College of Medicine from the University of Missouri intending to become a family doctor. He became interested in neuroscience and participated in the junior year neurology-neurosurgery clerkship and followed this with a neurosurgery elective. During the senior elective, I asked him to review the status of vasospasm in subarachnoid hemorrhage. Dick presented an excellent, lengthy, detailed review of the literature and told me that he wanted to train in neurosurgery. While clearing some office files last fall, I found a copy of that review. We have actually made strikingly little progress in the understanding and treatment of this condition since Dick Lister's paper. Several thousand papers have been published on the topic, in the interim, but the clinical solution still eludes us.

I initially suggested Dick consider training at Mayo Clinic, Minnesota, or Michigan, all good, sound Midwestern programs. I also recommended he consider the University of Florida, where Dr. Al Rhoton had just become chairman and was building a new neurosurgery department. New, rapidly developing departments often offer unrecognized opportunity. Dick was invited to stay at Dr. Rhoton's house, and was treated well by the small faculty and resident group. Dr. Rhoton offered him a place on Christmas Eve, and Dick became the first graduate of our school to enter neurosurgery residency.

The Neuroscience Department provided a third-year, six-week clerkship, during the first ten years of the medical school's existence. In that period, a student developed interest in neurology, neurosurgery, or neuroradiology virtually every year. This declined subsequently, with the elimination of the required junior year neuroscience clerkship. Students are overwhelmingly influenced by clerkship experiences of the third year. Most students have made a career decision as they enter the fourth year, making curriculum structure a determining factor in career choice. Medical schools offering clinical neuroscience in the third year consistently generate more candidates for neurological training.

Meeting and interviewing hundreds of students over the years, I found that a number of paths lead to a career caring for patients with neurological illness. Some become fascinated by the brain very early and pursue neuroscience in college. Some first become interested as the result of the neuroanatomy course in the first year of medical school and others are converted by an enthusiastic neurologist or neurosurgeon during their clinical clerkships.

A handful of American medical schools have a required

neuroscience clerkship in the third year and generate an inordinate number of clinical neuroscience physicians. Indiana University, Columbia Physicians and Surgeons, Harvard, Stanford, and the Johns Hopkins all have excellent undergraduate medical school experience in neuroscience and send numerous excellent candidates to residency programs. With the aging of America, increasing prevalence of degenerative neurological illness is creating a need to train substantially more neurologists. A 20% shortfall, projected by 2020, is not adequately appreciated by US academic medicine leadership. Medical school curriculum change is an essential requisite in addressing neurological care for our citizens.

A New Auctioneer: A Serious Post-Operative Problem

Jeff Able had been in serious pain for ten days, unable to sleep or lie flat. The pain had begun as he was driving the long road trip, back from auctioneering school in Texas. Jeff was a farmer who always wanted to be an auctioneer. He finally saved enough money to develop this new skill and was anxious to start. Jeff had pain deep in the right shoulder, radiating into his right arm, and his thumb felt numb, a typical compression of the 6th cervical nerve by a C5 C6 cervical disc rupture in his neck.

A cervical disc herniation can be operated from the front or the back of the neck. Each surgical approach has advantages and disadvantages. In the anterior approach, a transverse incision about 1 ½ inches long is made in the front of the neck and does not injure the musculature, resulting in a more comfortable postoperative experience. The posterior incision is longer and involves the deep neck muscles, is more painful after surgery, and the recovery is a bit longer. I had gradually done more of the acute cervical disc herniation operations anteriorly, for these reasons.

Myelography confirmed the diagnosis. I proceeded with surgery, performing it anteriorly with the microscope. This involved moving the larynx (voice box) to the side and pulling the muscle in front of the spine to the side with retractors. A large disc fragment was removed; the surgery proceeded rapidly and uneventfully. I went to see Jeff later in the day, and he was awake, and free of pain.

His voice was weak and very hoarse. This was worrisome with his new, beloved career! I rapidly went through each step in the operation, in my mind. The recurrent laryngeal nerve supplies the vocal cord, and lies between the larynx and esophagus. There are some anatomical variations that make it possible to injure or cut the nerve. The nerve supply to the vocal cord can be temporarily compressed with the retraction or pulling of the muscle. The inflated balloon on the tube in the windpipe for the anesthesia sometimes compresses the nerve and vocal cord. Voice change caused by nerve compression would be expected to recover in a few months while cutting the nerve would produce permanent change in voice.

I assured Jeff this was temporary and he would be in full voice in several months, demonstrating more confidence then I felt. At the scheduled 2-week post-surgery office visit, I entered the exam room hoping for the best. Jeff's voice was still weak and hoarse, no better and no worse. My worry continued and a one month visit was arranged. When I saw his name on the schedule the day before follow up, my worry began. At the office visit, he walked in beaming, his voice had returned rapidly, about a week before, and he was ready to auction!

Jeff's voice change was caused by transient compression from retraction, but an important lesson was learned. Always tailor the treatment precisely to the patient. Since voice was so important, an operation threatening his voice, even with a one to two percent risk, should not have been considered when another good solution, a posterior approach, existed. I did not offer him the choice as I should have, I made the decision. Given the facts, Jeff would have elected temporary discomfort avoiding risk to his new career. This was the first of a few voice complications experienced in anterior cervical spine surgery. The complication was well described in the literature and I had not done an adequate risk analysis. Risk analysis is a critical step in every operation and the physician owes the patient analysis and readily understood disclosure. I skipped that step, and learned a lesson, happily without lasting detriment to Jeff Able. I feel very fortunate that this happened rather early in my career, and I had the opportunity to learn without causing permanent injury to the patient.

Farming, My Other Occupation

Although bemused by Larry Holden's repeated trips to the dairy farm in upper New York State, I also had deep attachments to farming. My dad's occupation was managing a large tractor plant, and his major diversion was farming. He purchased his first farm in 1932 near Fairview in Fulton county, later in 1935, a small farm near Wyoming in Stark County, and finally, in 1937 an even smaller farm just outside of Morton in Tazewell county. During my high school years, he acquired a Mississippi river bottomland farm in a Levee district about 35 miles north of Saint Louis. He was a city boy fascinated by agriculture.

As a boy, I went to the farm frequently with Dad, where we raised corn, wheat, oats, and alfalfa hay. At Fairview, we raised pigs and cattle and I became familiar with the animals. At the time, the animals were cared for in a humane fashion in small numbers. There was nothing resembling a "factory farm" anywhere in the area. After WW II, we began to add soybeans to our corn, wheat, and clover crop rotation. Soybeans became important during WW II because access to vegetable oils from Asia had been cut. The farms steadily became more mechanized, less labor intensive, and less interesting.

The first years in Peoria I was totally occupied with developing neurology and neurosurgery in our hospitals and the College of Medicine. I lost Dad to esophageal cancer in 1974; I was immediately immersed in farming as I assumed his management role. On my trip to the Missouri farm, I drove through Bluffs on route 100 in Illinois, a tiny farm town with one stop sign and a bank that posted the price of corn, beans, and wheat. On one trip, there was a sign "Farm for Sale" that led me to the purchase of a bottom land farm behind a levee on the Illinois River. The farm was entirely flat and tillable; to my naïve eye, it looked perfect for raising corn and soybeans.

Laine Comerford had farmed the land for some time, and after we worked together a while, he was quite candid with me. He tended to use the word "quicksand" frequently in regard to some of the wet areas in the fields. He enthusiastically described losing a tractor in the "quicksand", and taking most of the day to retrieve it. With a sinking feeling, it became apparent to me that I was not an astute farmer or a judge of land. A few years, a great deal of drainage tile, and we gradually achieved a productive grain farm. In the spring, repeated rains brought worry about levee failure and flooding. Laine usually called late at night, to tell me that he was at the levee and the water was within 6 inches of the top of the levee, but the levee has held these past 40 years. We dealt with too much rain, too little rain, early frosts etc., and constant reminders of how little control man has over their environment.

Walking through soybeans or watching young pigs immediately removed the tensions of the hospital, clinic, and operating room. I stopped raising animals when factory farming arrived. Factory farming is inhumane and the whole process indefensible. I steadily became more troubled by how animals were cared for, in the pursuit of profit and competitively priced food. Over a relatively short time I became a vegetarian, first eliminating pork, then beef, then chicken from my diet. It was a simplistic emotional Don Quixote response, while continuing to grow large amounts of corn and soybeans, farm animal food. The soybeans can be used for cooking oil, and the corn can be converted to ethanol for auto fuel, one rationalization for continuing the status quo.

I still love to walk in the fields, especially in the spring and fall, providing a time of continuing reassessment. Yearly the costs for fertilizer and chemicals increase because of price escalation and increased chemical use. Manufacturers have insisted on the total safety of their products, but recently Roundup made by Monsanto has again been considered a possible human carcinogen. (1) We have used it as herbicide since the late '70s. Having considered the people that grew organic and those that insisted on organic products unrealistic, I am facing a late re-evaluation. I am progressively more skeptical of the intrinsic honesty of the American agricultural chemical industry. Our increasing use of agricultural chemicals potentially has a significant effect on population health, oncology, and human genetics. I have not attempted a conversion to organic farming. Large scale American grain farming will be very difficult to change and is totally dependent on insecticide, herbicide, and chemical fertilizers.

Chapter 6

Graduate Education: Neuroscience Residencies
A New Challenge and Opportunity
1979-2001

The direction in which education starts a man
will determine his future in life

—Plato

Developing Neurology and Neurosurgery Residencies

Although the immediate task was the development of the medical student program, the medical school had to develop graduate medical education (GME, residency and fellowship programs) and continuing medical education (CME) for practicing physicians if it were to change the quality of medical care in the Downstate. Studies show that doctors stay where they have graduate training. I participated in the University of Illinois committee structure supporting graduate medical education and ultimately chaired the graduate education committee on the Peoria Campus.

At the formation of the College of Medicine, the residencies were accredited to Saint Francis Hospital, except for the Family Medicine program at Methodist Hospital. The Saint Francis Hospital administration initially was reluctant to have the University involved in "their" programs. A critical decision was made rather early. The Family Practice residency would be sited at the Methodist Hospital in an "unopposed arrangement", no other residencies existed in that hospital. It was thought that family practice training thrived better in a hospital that did not have competing specialty residency programs. All other graduate programs were at Saint Francis Medical Center and later, the family medicine program at Saint Francis closed.

Ultimately a proposal for a University of Illinois neurology residency was developed in 1979 with Dr. Dennis Garwacki assuming the program directorship. Initially, we accepted one or two residents per year in neurology and general interest in the neurology residency was modest. A neurology residency was an essential step in building a comprehensive neurology department, and a basic requirement for establishing a neurosurgery residency. The neurology residency was the first graduate program to be accredited to the University rather than the hospital, an important milestone in the evolution of the College of Medicine.

The neurosurgery residency was provisionally approved in 1980, the first neurosurgery residency in a "branch" medical school in the United States. A number of academic neurosurgeons assured me we were unlikely to achieve approval of a new neurosurgery residency without a well established medical school. Invaluable support and advice were provided by Dr. Lyle French, chairman at the University of Minnesota and Dr. Sidney Goldring, Chairman at Washington University in Saint Louis. As a novice program director, I elected to begin the neurosurgery residency with a small cadre, taking one resident in alternate years. This was a mistake. I failed to appreciate the importance of fellow residents in the educational process.

Dr. William Olivero, a graduate of our medical school began July 1, 1981, as our first resident. Bill enjoyed pediatrics and neurosurgery. Subsequently, he pursued a pediatric neurosurgery fellowship after completing our program, continuing his interest in the care of children. We changed to one resident per year in a 6-year program almost immediately, and Jeffery Margetts came from the University of Utah as our second resident. At that time, the matching program in neurosurgery did not exist, and candidates were interviewed as they indicated interest. In Dr. Margetts' year, we interviewed three candidates, all staying at our Moss Avenue home. Gladys was impressed by Dr. Margetts because he made his bed neatly and the room was pristine. Jeff proved to be a hard working reliable resident.

The following year, Dr. Ali Niani asked to join our program because the Massachusetts General Hospital (MGH) program did not seem a good match for him. Ali had attended the Harvard Medical School and began training at the MGH. Ali worked hard, was original and creative, and added greatly to the program. Harvard's loss was our gain. At that point, I realized that in neurosurgery, where the number of faculty and residents are small and the program long, supportive interpersonal relationships are important in achieving individual potential. Dr. Patrick Tracy, who attended our medical school, was the fourth resident, after finishing 18 months of preliminary medicine and pediatrics. Dr. Dzung Dinh, who had attended medical school at the University of Iowa, came as our fifth resident, from the general surgery residency at Texas Southwestern. We had a full cadre for the first time.

Because our neurology program was in its early development, and a challenging neurology experience was essential, I explored several options to provide a strong neurology experience in the early days of the neurosurgery residency. At that time, the neurology residency at the University of California at San Francisco was one of the best in the United States. A visit to Dr. Robert Fishman, the chairman of the neurology department at UCSF, was my next step. After some discussion and visiting, Dr. Fishman agreed to take our resident for six months of neurology training, including one month of neuro-ophthalmology with Dr. Bill Hoyt, one of the world's leading experts in the field.

All was arranged, and Bill Olivero was the first to go to San Francisco. After several months, Bill told me it was a challenging experience and almost all his fellow neurology residents were M.D., Ph.D. graduates training to lead academic neurology careers. After five years, neurology at the University of Illinois had expanded significantly. The neurosurgery residents were able to do their entire residency on our campus, although a few left for 6-12 months research or specialty experience. The short relationship with Neurology at UCSF was invaluable, as the program developed.

Initially, the neurosurgery resident selection process was chaotic, with interviews occurring, and positions offered throughout the year. A few highly sought after centers required medical students to wait two or three years, after graduating, to begin their residency while other programs had open positions. The Society of Neurological Surgeons established a formal match process in 1983 that was set to begin in 1985. This allowed the residents and program faculty an opportunity to evaluate numerous options. Candidates visited multiple programs and both the candidate and the program faculty submitted a preference list, with the formal match occurring on a specific date.

Initially, there were rule violations by the candidates and the programs. Over the years, the match became a successful, transparent process with consistent adherence to regulations. Imperfections remain; candidates must interview at 10-20 programs to assure a place, an expensive and time-consuming process for the candidates and a significant workload for faculty. Academic neurosurgery has been ineffective in attempts to regionalize the interviews to decrease the time and cost for the medical students. Preliminary video interviews, Skype or other technology need exploration. Work on the match continues.

Creation of the neurosurgery residency was life-changing. In 1980, I still enjoyed virtually all aspects of operative neurosurgery, even the mundane details. I needed to assist as the residents learned to operate, and progressively give them independence and responsibility. After 20 years as an independent surgeon, this was a difficult transition to a new professional life. I was torn between providing the resident with a good experience and providing the patient more expert operative treatment from a senior neurosurgeon. A difficult struggle, never won. Throughout the remainder of my career, optimum delegation remained a challenge.

The other faculty were more effective in delegation of care and responsibility. This was particularly true as Drs. Olivero, Tracy, Dinh, and Lanzino joined the faulty and assumed the attending surgeon role. Over time, the problem was thus resolved compensating for my limitations. Both Dr. Cushing and Dr. Oldberg essentially never first assisted while a trainee operated. They apparently found assisting the trainee virtually impossible. I now understood their problem. I emulated Cushing and Oldberg in my failure to provide progressive delegation of responsibility. In recent years, the residency review committee for neurosurgery has assured residents achieve progressive clinical and operative independence.

The early days of the residency were painful, with important lessons learned slowly. The initial approval for the neurosurgery residency was provisional, with a site visit after two years. After this site visit, a letter arrived indicating the intent to withhold full accreditation. A number of sleepless nights followed. A fraction of the deficiency, as we identified, was a misunderstanding of the submitted data, and was then readily clarified. Other issues required substantive improvement in the program which was also accomplished. The second site visit was done by Dr. Bill Collins, the chairman at Yale. He was delightful, supportive, and provided valuable suggestions for improvement. The site visit resulted in full accreditation essentially free of difficulty in the ensuing years.

High quality education in neurological surgery is a team effort requiring support of multiple departments. The institution, at the time of the initial approval, was required to provide graduate education in surgery, medicine, neurology, and pediatrics. A full-time neuropathologist and neuroradiologist were specified and training in endocrinology, critical care, and neuro-anesthesia was expected. These requirements were more readily accomplished in large, established academic medical centers and demanded some team building and negotiation in Peoria. The neurosurgery residency was essential to the Level I trauma center designation, critical to the Mission of Saint Francis Medical Center. This need created strong institutional support to fulfill the requirements of the neurosurgery program. Fortunately, success was not dependent on my limited knowledge of team building.

The necessary infrastructure has increased with improving graduate education. The next challenge occurred in 1990, when the residency review committee added a radiology residency as a critical element. I immediately went to see Dr. Tom Cusack, the Head of the University radiology department, indicating we must have a radiology residency. The radiology department and the hospital immediately responded to the challenge. Dr. Terry Brady became the program director, more faculty were hired, and the first class of the radiology residency, taking 2 residents per year, started July 1, 1992, ultimately increasing to a complement of 4 residents per year.

A potential challenge developed in 2014, when consideration was given by the Neurosurgery Residency Review Committee (RRC) to the requirement of a residency program in anesthesiology. We did not have a residency in anesthesiology at the University of Illinois at Peoria. After further evaluation, the RRC continued with the expectation that adequate instruction in neuro-anesthesia is provided, and new programs must have an anesthesiology residency. Development of an anesthesia residency would bring an enhanced neuro-anesthesia program, entail further institutional commitment, and contribute to the research base of the program.

Residency programs are stronger, and systems are in place for continuous monitoring of activity assuring that residents avoid a lengthy period of inadequate education resulting from programmatic deficiencies. The University of Illinois neurosurgery residency has steadily improved, with greater surgery volumes, a larger faculty, and a greater variety of clinical challenges. The residency program now takes 2 residents, alternating with 1, per year in a seven-year program, with Dr. Klopfenstein as the department head and Dr. Julian Lin as the residency program director.

The residents now experience extensive spinal surgery instrumentation, deep brain stimulation, epilepsy surgery, congenital craniofacial anomaly surgery, brain tumor and pituitary surgery, and endovascular and microsurgical vascular surgery. We receive 200 applications for the 1 or 2 positions and interview 30 candidates. The residents learn much from their fellow residents, and the size and quality of the residency group is a major success factor. Recruitment of the best possible candidate is the most important step in building a program of sustained excellence. If the residents are exceptionally talented, they insist the program be excellent. The initial small cadre was an ill-advised misstep that should not occur in any new programs. Either have a moderately large, high-quality graduate program or eliminate the program.

Development of a neurology residency proved to be very challenging. The small department provided excellent clinical neurology care but lacked time and expertise to adequately support neurological graduate education. From the onset, the faculty was small and lacked members with research skills. Accreditation was lost in 1982. A new program was proposed in 1989, but accreditation was again withdrawn in 1997. The faculty was small and lacked essential subspecialists and faculty recruitment remained difficult. Lack of a neurology residency threatened the viability of the neurosurgery program. The program achieved re-accreditation in 1998 with the arrival and vigorous support of Dr. Jorge Kattah. Dr. Kattah recruited additional faculty, recruiting Drs. Sarah Zallek, Chris Zallek, and Greg Blume from the Methodist Medical Center of Illinois, thus adding neuromuscular and sleep medicine expertise to our neurology department. Dr. Meena Gujrati, who had joined in neuropathology, added a remarkable teaching presence to both the neurosurgery residency and the newly formulated neurology program. The neurology residency has steadily improved and grown in size, accepting 4 residents per year in a four-year program now led by program director Dr. Greg Blume. The residents work in a large stroke service, a comprehensive epilepsy center, and participate in other sub-specialty services. A large and gifted neurology faculty have developed an excellent experience for neurology residents. Both neurology and neurosurgery programs are developing a research infrastructure to support the career development of those joining the department.

The general goal is to know each resident well enough that the bar is set appropriately to assure optimum achievement. This entails a great deal of work and observation by the faculty. I fear we are only half way to that goal. Dr. Shroyer and Dr. Singh in 1951 at Bradley University demonstrated the importance of setting the bar, and how much work was involved to deliver the promise. This is the most important responsibility of the residency program director and University department head. Faculty must assist residents in developing habits that support clinical research, observation, discovery, and publication critical to a rewarding career free of "burn out".

Graduate education continues to undergo change, and the 80-hour work limitation required hospital leadership to develop an advanced practice nursing support system. Deborah Richardson, VP, COO of the Illinois Neurological Institute led the advanced practice nurse program to meet the challenge of sustained 24/7 patient care while supporting the educational mission of the graduate programs. Physicians in contemporary training programs learn to lead teams providing care, a change from their previous role as a solitary neurology consultant. The neurology and neuro-surgery residencies are constantly changing to prepare graduates to function in integrated health systems providing population and precision medicine. Neurologists and neurosurgeons will lead teams to provide the level of care expected while meeting quality and cost targets consistently. Together with primary care physicians, they develop care paths for investigation, a continuum of care, and effective care transitions. Administrative and clinical research skills will be addressed in evolving new residency programs.

Eighty percent of neurology residents take a specialty fellowship after completing residency. The University of Illinois neurology department will develop fellowships in vascular neurology, clinical neurophysiology, epilepsy, sleep, neurological critical care, multiple sclerosis, and movement disorders in the next ten years, to serve the population of the Midwest and to maintain a highly competitive residency program in neurology. Residents with great potential will match programs offering a spectrum of fellowship experiences.

Establishment of the seven-year neurosurgery program that may include a number of enfolded fellowships will diminish the demand for fellowships subsequent to the neurosurgery residency. The faculty continues to evaluate the value of fellowships in spinal neurosurgery, neurosurgical oncology, and cerebrovascular neurosurgery-microsurgery and endovascular surgery.

The aging of our population with increasing musculoskeletal problems is creating a need for more physiatrists to manage neck and back pain conservatively with fewer injections and interventions. The feasibility of a residency in physical medicine and rehabilitation requires further consideration. Rehabilitation is an important element of care in most forms of neurological illness. The absence of a graduate program in physical medicine and rehabilitation diminishes a team approach to education. A comprehensive neurological institute must include a sub-specialized physical medicine and rehabilitation program, responsive and integral to each specialized center. The INI has certified rehabilitation specialists in spine, stroke, neurological, and industrial rehabilitation. Faculty development to support a physical medicine and rehabilitation residency, accepting 2-4 residents per year, is a necessary next step.

Comprehensive neurological care is provided by an interdisciplinary team. Training the members of that team together is a necessary strategy. Residencies and fellowships in neurology, neurosurgery, vascular neurology, neurological critical care, diagnostic neuroradiology, interventional neuroradiology, neuropathology, physical medicine and rehabilitation, neuropsychology, and anesthesia all reinforce each other. This is a strong argument for planning the entire educational spectrum in the portfolio.

Graduate education is adjusting to a shortened patient length of stay, an 80 hour work week, a shift to outpatient care, and transparent cost and quality data. The more contemplative, research-oriented, scholarly world of outstanding academic centers of the '50, and '60s era is gone. We struggle to educate physicians who will generate new and disruptive treatments while avoiding a shift mentality and loss of humanity. With the dramatic increase in medical knowledge, our educational processes have to become much more efficient. Kenneth Ludmerer discusses the challenges in graduate education, of the past 20 years, in his book *Let Me Heal.* (1) He explores changes that should inspire young clinicians to continually address America's needs.

MRI Scanning:
The Second Revolution Progresses

In 1983, clinical Magnetic Resonance Imaging (MRI) became available, and Saint Francis Medical Center obtained a 0.5 Tesla Siemens magnet, the first installed in Illinois. MRI greatly enhanced the quality of anatomical imaging of the brain. The initial machines had a small aperture limiting the imaging function to the head. Dr. Robert Wright was so intrigued that he discontinued performing cerebral angiography, delegating this to others. He devoted his time to explore what could be accomplished with this paradigm-changing advance. He devised specialized coils, working with University of Illinois and Siemens engineers to generate better images. There was great interest in MRI on the Urbana Champaign campus (UIUC). Dr. Paul Lauterbur, a faculty member at UIUC shared the Nobel Prize in Medicine in 2003 with Peter Mansfield for fundamental research leading to the development of clinical MRI. We were involved in studying cutting-edge imaging, but we were publishing only a few case reports from our clinical service.

The next step was an increase in the size of the aperture of the scanner, thus permitting scans of the body. The technology could now be utilized for evaluation of spinal problems. This evolution was virtually the same as experienced with CT scanning ten years earlier. Over several years image quality was refined with the first application for spinal tumor, but ultimately with improving resolution, MRI was utilized to evaluate discogenic disease and spondylosis and the need for myelography dropped precipitously.

In 1988, Gadolinium was approved as a contrast agent to enhance tumor visualization in MRI, a further improvement in precise anatomical visualization without invasive testing. Gadolinium had paramagnetic properties that made it very visible on MRI. A chelated organic compound of Gadolinium was taken up by tumors enhancing the information provided by imaging. The second major revolution in clinical neuroscience, precision imaging, had gradually evolved with CT in 1973, then MRI in 1983. High field magnets and improved imaging sequences yielded incremental improvement over the next 30 years. Diagnosis became immensely easier in a relatively short time allowing one to plan surgery in detail before the operation, decreasing patient discomfort and complications.

The MRI imaging revolution evolves with each decade bringing increasing ability to image white matter pathways in the brain, nuclear anatomy, and brain function. With biomarkers, imaging is contributing to the understanding of some of the unconquered degenerative diseases. The strength of the magnets has steadily increased over the years since our first 0.5 Tesla (T) magnet. Clinical magnets now operate at 3 T, and 7 T, and higher strength magnets are becoming commonplace for research studies, in academic health centers. More powerful magnets, and improved coils and imagining programs have increased complexity and imaging capability. OSF SFMC added an MRI Physicist, Wen-Ching Liu, Ph.D., to the staff, thus recognizing the critical importance of these developments in clinical care and research in neurological disease.

MRI is now being used for direct targeting of nuclei in the thalamus during stereotactic surgery for Parkinson's disease. Some centers are now doing Deep Brain Stimulator placement under general anesthesia without physiological testing, utilizing MRI anatomical targeting. A significant trend in intraoperative MRI guided stereotactic surgery for small deep brain lesions and epilepsy surgery is developing in large centers. A two room suite was installed at Saint Francis Medical Center to perform MRI guided neurosurgery in January 2016.

Botulism Strikes in Peoria:
Neurological Intensive Care Unit

October 14, 1983, a 25-year-old man arrived in the emergency room at Saint Francis Medical Center complaining of shortness of breath, seeing double, and his legs were heavy. Within 30 minutes, an older woman arrived with similar complaints. Dr. John Ruthman, the attending physician in the emergency room, made the uncommon diagnosis of botulism, rarely seen in the United States. Botulism is a serious, often fatal paralytic illness caused by a toxin produced by Clostridium botulinum. The toxin affects the neuromuscular junction resulting in paralysis and respiratory failure. Some characteristics mimic other neurological illness, but the arrival of several patients, in a short time span, clarified the problem. Over the weekend, 28 patients were admitted and seen by Dr. Stephen Doughty, infectious disease attending physician, and his team. Treatment involved anti-toxin and meticulous supportive care. A portion of the patients needed respiratory assistance almost immediately. All had a "patty melt" sandwich with sautéed onions at the Skewer Inn in the local shopping mall. (1) The Center for Disease Control (CDC) subsequently, proved the sautéed onions to be the source of botulism. This was the third largest botulism outbreak reported in the United States, since 1899.

The new neurological ICU was opened immediately that weekend, a week before the planned opening. We were not ready, but we reacted rapidly, with the unit filling with patients requiring respirators. Our new unit was one of the early dedicated neurological intensive care units in the Midwest and represented a substantial improvement in care. It allowed our nursing staff to acquire expertise in acute neurological illness with concentration of their experience. We added experienced staff who worked extraordinary hours; patients and their families received dedicated care and all survived. We never had the planned grand opening, substituting a trial by fire that immediately demonstrated the value of the neurological intensive care unit.

Neurological critical care units developed as distinct entities from general or surgical ICU's in the mid-to-late '70s, with a large academic unit opening at the Massachusetts General Hospital in 1977. An earlier twelve-bed unit had opened in the Mayo Clinic in 1958. These were all initially "open units" meaning the patients were cared for by their attending neurologist or neurosurgeon. With increasing size of the service at Saint Francis Medical Center and development of a neurology and neurosurgery residency, a neurological intensive care unit was needed. I began discussions with hospital leadership and Sue Wozniak, the chief nursing officer. They agreed that the need existed and we planned a twelve-bed unit by converting part of a third-floor nursing unit. A nursing staff was trained. Our timing fortuitously prepared us for the botulism outbreak.

Later we acquired a large 24-bed unit on the third floor allowing development of an intensive care unit integrated with an adjacent intermediate care unit. This geographic continuity allowed a seamless transition of care as the patient's status improved. Patients and families experienced less disruption with the "hand off" to the next level of care. Patients acutely ill were admitted to the neurological intensive care unit, with improvement moved within the unit to an intermediate care bed, and then graduated to the acute neurology unit, all on the same floor. This avoided confusion for families, and allowed nurses to see the recovery of patients and the course of their illness. The opportunity increased nursing skills and made work fulfilling. Adjacent related ICU, intermediate, and acute care units do provide a sound model for the continuum of care. This specialized neurological care model requires nursing expertise not supported by less specialized cross coverage units. Large units with consistent occupancy are required for this model to be economically feasible. After a number of years, hospital leadership moved the neurological ICU to a floor with other ICU units, separating it from the intermediate and acute care facility.

In the early years, the patients in neurological ICU were cared for by their neurosurgeons or neurologists. The development of physician specialization in neurological critical care came later. Seven neurologists from a number of leading medical centers took the first step to form a national neuro-critical care society in 1999. Over time subspecialty accreditation and certification occurred. Neurological ICU's are now staffed by specialists consistently present in the units.

Neurological critical care units are staffed by a variety of internists, neurologists, anesthesiologists, and neurosurgeons with specialized skills in critical care. The United Council for Neurologic Subspecialties developed a training and accreditation program for Neurocritical Care for neurologists seeking a critical care career. Initially, this examination was taken by neurologists and internists trained in critical care medicine. Neurosurgeons have, as a specialty, become interested in critical care medicine and milestones were incorporated in the neurosurgery residency program. The Society of Neurological Surgeons Committee for Advanced Subspecialty Care (CAST) developed a fellowship and certification program for neurosurgeons wishing to subspecialize in neurological critical care, and critical care became an integral part of the neurosurgical residency training.

Some units are managed as "open" units with the patient's physician able to write orders and participate in care. Other units are "closed" with management and orders done by the attending intensivist. Management decisions are more timely with this change in physician staffing, but the potential for failure in communication is increased. All of these staffing variations continue to be evaluated; a definitive optimum state remains to be identified. Several years ago, OSF HealthCare added eICU oversight that provides centralized monitoring of all ICU patients 24/7, adding another layer of surveillance to the patient care process. The overall effect has been substantive progress in the critical care of patients suffering neurological illness. Fine tuning of the process continues.

The Society of Neurological Surgeons and Neurosurgical "Clubs"

Walking down the hall at the Johns Hopkins Hospital in 1987, a neurosurgical physician acquaintance congratulated me. Later I found I had been elected to the Society of Neurological Surgeons.

It was a long wait, starting with my invitation as a guest in 1980, at the San Francisco meeting hosted by the University of California. The national association for academic faculty in neurosurgery, the "Senior Society", was founded as the Society of Neurological Surgeons (SNS) in 1920, and is the oldest neurosurgical association in the world.

A candidate generally is elected to the rather small membership on the basis of their career as a neurosurgical educator, leader, or investigator, and the durability of their academic program. When first invited, I was puzzled and felt a decided outsider, coming in from the country, not an academician, and clearly not from an established department. The membership of the Senior Society apparently agreed because, although I continued as an invited guest, I was not elected to membership until the 1987 meeting at Johns Hopkins Hospital. This was the first indication that our nascent program might endure. It was now necessary to purchase a tuxedo to attend the annual formal dinner of the Society.

After 38 years of attending the Senior Society meeting, I am a "senior" member of the "Senior Society" and comfortable in my role. I attend annually because, unlike the other large neurosurgical associations, at the SNS meeting, I can find my friends and get invaluable advice. Topics that are important to those responsible for leading academic departments are considered, and ideas and excitement regarding the future abound. The first day of the annual meeting, the program director's day, is devoted entirely to change and improvement in the neurosurgery residency training programs. There is intense interest in the educational process and helping develop educational and research infrastructure. The second day of the meeting is devoted to the work of the host department. The annual meeting, over time, has given me the opportunity to visit the major neurosurgery departments in the United States. The remaining day and a half is devoted to new developments in neuroscience. Membership in this group has been helpful in my struggle to create a department. Each year it has given me renewed enthusiasm for building the academic program. I always return with a long list of "to do" that I am sure is a recurring annoyance to my colleagues.

The Harvey Cushing Society was founded in 1931 as a venue for younger neurosurgeons who were not members of the SNS. Virtually each neurosurgical "club" was founded by those who failed to be admitted to a more senior club. The first meeting of the Harvey Cushing Society was in Boston in 1932 with 23 people in attendance. My mentor, Dr. Eric Oldberg, was one of the founding members. This new club honored Harvey Cushing, who had retired from the Brigham Hospital. The Cushing Society required members to be board certified, after formation of the Board in 1942. New research work was presented at the annual meeting of this group in the early days of neurosurgery, making attendance important. Early on, a large part of the membership was trained by Dr. Cushing. The Society name was changed in 1967 to the American Association of Neurological Surgeons (AANS) because most of the members no longer were in the Cushing linage. The Society assumed a role representing neurosurgery nationally. Fortunately, I became a member in time to have the Harvey Cushing Society on my certificate.

The Congress of Neurological Surgeons was founded in 1951 with 121 members at the first meeting and its goal was primarily the education of young members. Board certification was not required, the meeting occurred in the fall, and there was less emphasis on research. The Congress adapted education of their members as their niche with less emphasis on evolving science.

The two major neurosurgery groups, the Congress of Neurological Surgeons (meeting in the fall) and the American Association of Neurological Surgeons (meeting in the spring) have become similar as the years pass. The attendance is so large that it is difficult to find professional friends and acquaintances. There is an unfortunate tendency to utilize the same speaker on repetitive topics from year to year. Over the years, the two organizations have both become quite large and duplicative and their annual meetings involve massive commercial support from Pharma, instrument makers, and other vendors. The AANS has gone from a meeting with 23 in attendance, for several days, to a 4-day meeting attended by 4500 or more, a significant change in the "neurosurgical club", since I entered.

New work is often presented at AANS/CNS subspecialty meetings. Each society has attendance requirements for members, resulting in a duplicative effort and appreciable expense for the individual neurosurgeon. In a day of mounting concern regarding the cost of medical care, serious consideration is building for a merger of the two organizations. A large number of the neurosurgeons support this, but the officers of the respective organizations and their administrators are in opposition. This is an interesting study in conservative organizational leadership behavior.

The organizations are not addressing the change in their role possible with evolving communication technology. Both organizations have failed to respond to progress in digital communication, decreasing the need for prolonged on-site national meetings. Just as the physical structure and function of the medical library have changed in a digital world, the national meetings will inevitably evolve with technological change. The organizations will undoubtedly evolve more slowly than available technology, with physicians continuing to travel to meetings, failing to make optimum use of communication technology

The Third Revolution

The third revolution, image-guided neurosurgery evolved step-wise over many years, with our faculty participating from the outset. Creation of digital information with CT or MRI scanning, with increasingly inexpensive computing power, led to the development of surgery directed by data derived from these digital images. Surgery was no longer dependent on the limits of human vision. The era when I looked at a seemingly normal brain, and attempted to estimate where the culprit was hiding under the surface, was over. MRI images taken before surgery direct us to a dime-sized tumor deep in the brain, thus avoiding injury to critical structures on the way.

The revolution began simply with a frame providing three-dimensional coordinate measurements attached to the skull and imaging from the CT scanner to direct a brain probe. The probe was used to create a brain lesion with radiofrequency heat or obtain a piece of tumor for biopsy purposes. In the late '70s the Brown-Roberts-Wells (BRW), then a Cosman-Roberts Wells (CRW) frame were developed at the University of Utah. This frame made the process simple enough that multiple centers rapidly applied the technology. Dr. Lister led the development of the stereotactic brain biopsy program, on his return from the University of Florida in 1980.

Computer power became cheaper and faster, and imaging of the brain improved dramatically with the advent of MRI, permitting precise targeting. If image guidance was to be utilized widely, it had to escape the constraints of the stereotactic frame. Dr. Bucholz in Saint Louis in 1993, utilized an optical digitizer and Light Emitting Diode(LED) equipped instruments to relate operative localization with preoperative images. The light emitted from the handle of the instrument was recorded by digitizers, in the line of sight in the room, and the computer systems related that to the MRI images recorded before surgery. The result; the tip of the instrument related to the preoperative images providing precise guidance without the limitations of a frame. The surgeon knew where the tip of the instrument was in relation to the brain. This work was ultimately developed into the commercially available

Stealth Station by Medtronic.

Craniotomies are now performed with the guidance of pre-operative MRI images. Over time, more data has been obtained from the MRI imaging sequences, visualizing the white matter pathways in the brain, allowing us to avoid damage to these structures as tumors, blood vessel abnormalities, and blood clots are approached and removed. All of this was readily applied to the brain, because unlike the heart and lungs, the skull does not move. On a micro basis, we were finding our way through the brain very much like people use GPS in their automobile to find a house in an unfamiliar city. The patient's MRI is used to develop guidance similar to a Google map system, leading the surgeon to the target.

The brain does shift after some of the cerebrospinal fluid is removed during surgery, diminishing the accuracy of the guidance. BrainLab, a German firm with software expertise entered the neuronavigation market in 1989, ultimately leading to Brain Suite development incorporating intraoperative MRI, in 2004. The neurosurgery department's next step in image guided surgery was an operating room equipped with an MRI scanner that allows for patients undergoing procedures to be moved into the magnet for a progress check. This step eliminated the inaccuracy created with brain movement. Some less complex procedures can be done within the confines of the magnet.

A two-room intraoperative MRI suite was opened in January 2016. A 3 T imaging magnet is located in a room adjacent to the operative suite. After a portion of the tumor operation is completed, the patient is moved into the MRI and images obtained, then the patient is returned to the OR for further surgery or incision closure. The MRI unit is used for diagnostic imaging of other patients, when not active with surgery. Additional applications of surgery performed within the magnet are in the research stage; laser ablation of tumors and epileptogenic foci, and direct targeting for deep brain stimulation electrode placement.

Because the spine is made up of articulated segments allowing movement between segments, the move to image guidance proceeded more slowly for spinal surgery. Medtronic developed an O Arm machine that allows an intraoperative CT scan of the spine to be utilized for guidance in the placement of pedicle screws and other procedures in complex spinal reconstructive surgery. Dr. Fassett initiated the spinal guidance program in early 2014. BrainLab and other companies are developing systems for image guidance in spine surgery. This development decreases surgical time and cost of reconstructive surgery while improving quality and safety. The screws and instrumentation to make the spine stable can now be placed with computer-supported precision.

The Third Revolution led to more precise surgery in the brain and spine with smaller exposures, less blood loss, shorter operative times, and less damage to normal structures.

Radiosurgery with Linac and Gamma Knife

Lars Leksell developed radiosurgery in Sweden, delivering a single high dose of radiation to a precise location in the brain. Leksell was initially interested in relief of trigeminal neuralgia facial pain. He developed the Gamma Knife, a multisource radioactive Cobalt 60 machine producing focused photon radiation. Early on, the imaging was too poor for precise targeting of the radiation. An insightful concept awaiting the right technology for clinical application in patients. In 1975 improved targeting with brain CT images made the Gamma Knife useful. Great precision in cranial radiosurgery awaited the development of MRI imaging in the mid-'80s.

Ladislau Steiner from Karolinska Hospital, Stockholm repeatedly brought results of his radiosurgical obliteration of brain arteriovenous malformations to US neurosurgery meetings. I was initially skeptical of his reported results, fearing that he was publishing only his successful cases. Dr. Dade Lunsford, after completing neurosurgical training at the University of Pittsburgh, visited and worked with the radiosurgery team in Stockholm. In 1987, the University of Pittsburgh Medical Center (UPMC) installed the first Gamma Knife in the United States. The following year, I invited Dr. Lunsford as a visiting professor to the University of Illinois Neurosurgery Department, a first step in developing radiosurgery. Meanwhile, further reports suggested that stereotactic radiosurgery was an important neurosurgical advance. Shortly thereafter, Dr. Steiner moved from Stockholm's Karolinska Institute to the University of Virginia and installed the second US Gamma Knife there.

My visit to the University of Virginia was convincing; we must develop a radiosurgery program. A proposal to purchase a Gamma Knife, an expenditure of $ 3 million was presented to Saint Francis Medical Center leadership. They understandably felt the cost structure was prohibitive, and offered to commit $500,000 to develop a method utilizing our radiation therapy linear accelerator for radiosurgery. We would use our Cosman-Roberts-Wells (CRW) stereotactic frame for targeting. Although other US centers were utilizing this method, I was uncomfortable with the compromise, feeling the precision of the Gamma Knife was superior.

We did proceed with the linear accelerator as our radiation source, to avoid falling far behind in an important new field. In 1990, we began to treat small numbers of AVM's, acoustic tumors, and skull base meningiomas with radiosurgery using the linear accelerator. The treatment was a long difficult process with application of the frame early in the day, followed by treatment planning MRI and CT. Working with the physicist, we planned much of the day and administered the treatment in the early evening, when the linear accelerator became available. The accelerator was used all day to treat cancer patients. The result was a long day for patients who needed to wear the stereotactic frame for twelve hours. I worked with Dr. Jim McGee and Dr. Brian Griffin, radiation oncologists, and Greg Devanna, physicist, during this prolonged process.

In 2000, with growth of the service, it was feasible to obtain a Model C Gamma Knife and an active program was rapidly built to serve patients in downstate Illinois. We were treating vestibular schwannoma (tumor on nerves of hearing and balance), arteriovenous malformations (AVMs), meningiomas, trigeminal neuralgia, and metastatic tumors. Treatment of each represented a change in management requiring culture change by the referring physicians. Radiosurgery was not a widely recognized treatment. Multiple visits around the state accomplished the transformation, and we were functioning at the international state of the art in radiosurgery.

The most striking change was in small vestibular tumors and small deep arteriovenous malformations. Both were often discovered when the symptoms were minimal or mild and established treatment required long complex operations. We arranged patient's clinic visits in the afternoon. The following morning, a frame was applied painlessly with local anesthesia. An MRI was done, a plan developed, and treatment given. In patients with AVM, a cerebral angiogram was also required. The patient returned home later that day and to work in several days, rather than spending days in the hospital, and being away from work for weeks. Gamma Knife radiosurgery, over ten years, became a major tool in the neurosurgery department.

In 2007, the Gamma Knife Cobalt-60 radiation sources had exhausted their half-life, treatment times were long, and fresh radiation sources were necessary. Cobalt-60 has a half- life of 5.26 years; at that point the treatment took twice as long as in 2000. A new Leksell machine had been developed; the "PerfeXion", and we elected to obtain the second machine in the Midwest. Mayo

Clinic had received theirs several months earlier. The patient no longer had to come out of the machine at each step in the treatment (a "shot") to allow us to manually reset the coordinates on the frame, as required with the Model C. The machine reset the coordinates with a mechanized helmet driven by the computer planning program, speeding treatment. The new program permitted precise delivery of radiation, sparing the adjacent structures more than previously possible.

My instruction in use of the PerfeXion unit was done at Hôpital de la Timone, Marseille, France. The manufacturer, Eleckta, installed the first worldwide PerfeXion machine there under the direction of Dr. Jean Regis. The French medical system concentrates specialty care, and Hôpital de la Timone had two Gamma Knife units and did the radiosurgery for a large part of France as well as some international referrals. Treating 8-10 patients each day yielded extensive experience in a short time, an excellent learning experience. Dr. Regis maintained meticulous, long-term treatment records.

The service at Hôpital de la Timone is an excellent example of development of new clinical knowledge through thoughtful analysis of meticulous clinical records. Dr. Regis has published multiple papers describing the technique and results in virtually every condition managed by radiosurgery. The cost in Cobalt based radiosurgery is largely determined by the cost of the apparatus. The radiation sources steadily decay, irrespective of the volume of patients receiving treatment. The French healthcare system is economical; a machine is used for eight to ten patients per day while in many US installations, one to three patients are treated each day. The geographic centralization of French specialty services would be unacceptable to American patients or physicians.

The PerfeXion allowed us to treat multiple metastatic tumors rapidly, avoiding radiation to the whole brain. Whole brain radiation does result in the development of dementia in some patients after 18 to 24 months. PerfeXion has also permitted administration of higher doses to small radio-resistant tumors such as renal cell and colon carcinoma. As the systemic treatment of the primary cancer has improved, patients sometimes live many years, and this new method of protecting brain function is an important advance in cancer treatment.

As my role as an administrator of the Illinois Neurological Institute required more time commitment, it was apparent that it was appropriate to transition my role in radiosurgery. Dr. Jeff Klopfenstein began to see new patients and do the treatment planning. I formally left the radiosurgery clinic in October 2013, after 24 years of participating in each step of radiosurgery development. Leaving the Gamma Knife Center was as difficult as giving up aneurysm and AVM surgery years earlier. Radiosurgery had transformed the care of small deep blood vessel abnormalities, vestibular tumors, and some metastatic cancer. It is being studied in multiple centers for the treatment of some seizure disorders, movement disorders (Parkinson's disease), and obsessive- compulsive disorders and there is exciting potential for further development.

Brain Tumor Surgery: "In and Out"

Tim Short, a 31-year-old accountant was curious; did he have a serious problem? He had intermittent buzzing in his right ear for three months that initially seemed to come and go, but recently was consistently present. This morning, while walking to his desk, he suddenly became dizzy and almost fell. The episode cleared, but his wife felt a visit to the doctor was necessary. Two weeks later the buzzing remained and he saw his physician. A brain MRI was ordered and performed two weeks later. After another week, the doctor's nurse called "you have a brain tumor".

Consultation with a neurosurgeon was arranged in a city near his home. He received the news he had a vestibular schwannoma 10 mm in size, in the base of his brain, that would require surgery. This was a small, slowly growing, benign tumor the size of a large pea on the nerve responsible for balance and next to nerves for facial movement and hearing. He was warned there was some possibility of facial weakness and he would almost certainly lose hearing in the right ear. The surgery would take four to five hours, he would be hospitalized for four to five days, and he would be away from work for three to four weeks.

His wife was uncomfortable with the advice offered and searched the internet to review the treatment of Tim's condition. She concluded Gamma Knife treatment was possible and asked Tim to consider further consultation. He was seen in the INI Radiosurgery clinic later that week, and treatment scheduled. At that time, tumors of this size had been treated with Gamma Knife in Sweden for almost 20 years with control rates in the 95 percent range, with 60-70 percent preservation of hearing and no facial weakness.

Tim arrived at 5:30 in the morning and after mild sedation, two points in the forehead and two points in the back of the head were numbed with local anesthetic, and a Leksell frame attached to his skull with four screws. Measurement strips on the Leksell frame were visualized on the MRI scan for localization purposes. The MRI images were utilized to plan the treatment of the tumor. Radiation was delivered to multiple discrete areas in the tumor, each touching the other, delivering 12 Gy of radiation to the entire tumor. The computer planning and imaging were so precise that the dose to the adjacent cochlea of the inner ear was less than 4 Gy. We knew from the experience at the University of Pittsburgh that the possibility of long-term preservation of hearing was excellent at this cochlear dose. Tim was placed on the couch of the Gamma Knife, the frame attached to the mechanism of the machine, and treatment was delivered, taking about 90 minutes. After treatment to each area, the couch, directed by the computer, moved the head to the next target area driven by computer coordinates. At completion of the planned treatment, the frame was removed, and he returned home and then to work in several days. In the years following, the tumor shrunk about 10 percent, has not grown or caused further symptoms, and his right ear hearing has remained good. He still has some intermittent buzzing.

In many respects, Tim's story is indicative of a trend in medicine; decreasing invasiveness in treatment. In earlier years, he would have a very painful pneumoencephalogram (air study) to demonstrate the tumor. This study would only be done after the tumor was a good deal larger because it was such a formidable experience. Tests of this magnitude were not done until the symptoms were severe enough to warrant invasive testing. In my early days in Peoria, vestibular schwannomas were often the size of an egg, when first diagnosed. Surgery for these very large tumors took eight to ten hours and often, was associated with at least partial permanent facial paralysis. Surgery always resulted in the loss of any remaining hearing.

Early in my life as a brain surgeon, surgery for vestibular schwannoma was a favorite operation. The operation was technically demanding, a cure was often achieved, and it was a challenge. The advent of the Gamma Knife rendered this technical feat unnecessary. A patient's decreased pain and disability is more rewarding.

Chapter 7

Illinois Neurological Institute 2001-2008

The brain is the organ of destiny, it holds within its humming mechanism secrets that will determine the future of the human race.

—Wilder Penfield

The Illinois Neurological Institute

A Neurological Institute, a collection of clinicians and scientists caring for people, improving care, and achieving a new understanding of the nervous system remained my vision after visiting Montreal Neurological Institute and The Neurological Institute of New York in 1957. Exposure to Dr. Percival Bailey and his experience in Paris enhanced my interest in the history of the development of neurology. There was a rich history of commitment to understanding the brain in many neurological institutes in Europe and America.

Percival Bailey introduced me to the history of neurological care in France. In 1654, Louis XIV charged architect Liberal Bruant to build a hospital, Hospice de la Salpetriere on the grounds of a gunpowder factory. Between 1785 and 1826, Pinel developed a center for psychiatric care at the Salpetriere. Jean-Martin Charcot became director of clinics in 1862 and developed Neurology, dealing with epilepsy, neurosyphilis, and stroke. Charcot developed original descriptions of amyotrophic lateral sclerosis and multiple sclerosis.

The first chair in neurology in the world was created for Charcot in 1882. Babinski became department head following Charcot in 1895 and encouraged the development of neurosurgery by Thierry de Martel and Clovis Vincent. The Hôpital de la Pitie was moved next to the Salpetriere in 1911, establishing the Pitie-Salpetriere as a large general hospital in Paris containing the largest neurological institute in Europe. Several years ago, I visited the services in a fully integrated Babinski building, a neurological hospital within the largest 2100 bed general hospital in Paris. I felt I was retracing Dr. Bailey's travels so many years before. The clinical services are associated with neuroscience research groups in neurobiology, neurochemistry, neuropharmacology, neurogenetics, neuroimmunology, and neurophysiology under the auspices of the French National Research Institutes. These laboratories are located in a research institute adjacent to the Babinski clinical building. The French approached neurological specialty care like they targeted other national problems, with centralization and specialization, unacceptable to the American people. (2) In a recent visit, I was struck by the product of the French commitment to centralization, while at the same time, preserving their history. The Chapelle de la Salpetriere, Liberal Bruant's masterpiece built in 1675 still stands and functions on the hospital grounds.

The English also addressed neurological care early. The National Hospital at Queen Square, founded in London in 1859, is now the National Hospital for Neurology and Neurosurgery (NHNN), a 244-bed unit integrated with University College London Hospitals since 1996. After opening, neurologists Brown-Sequard, Gowers, Hughlings Jackson, and neurosurgeon Victor Horsley contributed to Queen Square becoming a world destination for those seeking neurological diagnosis and care. With the advent of the National Health Service (NHS) and the integration of the National Hospital with University College London Hospitals and the NHS, the NHNN assumed a role in neurological population health and is a destination for the complex care of rare neurological illness in the United Kingdom. NHNN has 22 neurosurgeons and over 100 neurologists on staff, with graduate training programs in all neurological specialties and an extensive clinical and laboratory research program. The National Health Service has centralized and regionalized specialty neurological care, in a fashion different from the French, but with a good deal of centralization. (3)

The Neurological Institute of New York (NINY) was founded in 1909, by neurologists Joseph Collins, Joseph Fraenkel, and Pierce Bailey. Neurosurgeon Charles Elsberg saw patients requiring surgery. The Neurological Institute joined Columbia Presbyterian

Medical Center in 1925 and moved to the 168th Street campus, occupying a 14 story 191-bed hospital integrated with the Presbyterian hospital. This hospital has been led by neurologists Houston Merritt and Lewis Rowland and neurosurgeons J. Lawrence Pool, Ben Stein, and Robert Solomon. From the founding, neurologists have played a significant role in the design and execution of the mission. The NINY gradually developed all of the supporting specialties, and a graduate education and research program. The NINY is now integrated into a multi-hospital healthcare delivery system in metropolitan New York. Patient care is housed in the Milstein Building in the general hospital, and the original NINY building is a research and education facility. There are multiple neurological centers in Manhattan, demonstrating the stunning diversity and competitive approach taken in the United States. (4)

Wilder Penfield, a neurosurgeon at the NINY, wished to develop a neurological institute that incorporated fundamental research in brain function with clinical care. In 1932, the Rockefeller Foundation provided $ 1.2 million for construction and endowment. The City of Montreal and the Provence of Quebec provided additional support. Thus, the Montreal Neurological Institute (MNI) was designed and built as a hospital within Royal Victoria Hospital, a teaching hospital of McGill University. Penfield recruited neurology, EEG, neuropsychology, neuroradiology, and neurochemistry staff to form an institution committed to clinical care while furthering the understanding of nervous system function. Wilder Penfield neurosurgeon, Herbert Jasper electoencephalographer, and Brenda Milner neuropsychologist made fundamental discoveries regarding seizure disorders and brain function. K.A.C. Elliott, Professor of Neurochemistry identified gamma aminobutyric acid (GABA) as the first inhibitory neurotransmitter.

The MNI continues to be a center recognized for epilepsy research, brain imaging, cognitive neuroscience, neuroimmunology, and complex neural systems. The MNI may ultimately be incorporated in a large new McGill University Teaching Hospital currently being constructed. At present, it continues as a distinct entity in its historical facility. The MNI is probably somewhat less unique in Canada now than at its inception because of the development of a vigorous center in Toronto and the increasingly French character of the Provence of Quebec. (5)

My trip to Fargo, North Dakota in November 1968 demonstrated the full spectrum of facilities from rather modest to grand that might be developed. In 1977, after reviewing the development of the Barrow Neurological Institute by Dr. John Green in Phoenix, it seemed time to explore this concept in Peoria. John had finished neurosurgical training with Dr. Oldberg after WW II. Because of illness with rheumatic fever and arthritis, he sought a warm, dry climate. Dr. Green was the first neurosurgeon in Arizona, a pioneer. He was interested in epilepsy after working with Fred Gibbs and Percival Bailey at the NPI and was influenced by Wilder Penfield. The husband of one of his brain tumor patients, Charles Barrow, made a substantial donation, and with the support of Saint Joseph Hospital, the Barrow Neurological Institute opened in 1962. It seemed an appropriate model, of modest size and located within Saint Joseph Hospital.

In 1977, I talked with Mr. Ed McGrath, the associate administrator of Saint Francis Hospital Medical Center concerning a neurological institute within Saint Francis. I designed a four floor 100-bed inpatient facility with an outpatient clinic on the first floor. Neuroradiology and surgery were planned for the second floor, and the inpatient facilities occupied the 3rd and 4th floors. The proposed site was the open land on Glen Oak between the hospital and the Interstate highway immediately adjacent to the general hospital. Ed was puzzled, taken aback perhaps, but interested and proposed a visit to Barrow.

We arrived in Phoenix in mid-summer. The door to the plane was opened and a stairway moved to exit the aircraft. We were struck by hot wind and sand, my first trip to the desert! Dr. Green had developed a neurological specialty hospital within Saint Joseph Hospital, had residents in training, and had a modest research program. It was a fruitful trip; this was something we could do in Peoria! We returned, had a positive visit with Bill Franklin, President of Caterpillar, and began to think in terms of fundraising, and moving ahead with a building.

It was a time of periodic reassessment in medicine. There was a developing national consensus that medical care would significantly move to the outpatient arena. Both Ed and I were concerned that we were creating 100 potentially unnecessary beds in the community and mutually lost courage. We would work with the facilities we had, a neurological institute would not be built. This was an opportunity lost and a mistake. (1)

After a few years, the residencies were developing, and progress continued as a neurological center. We based the fifth year of the neurosurgery residency at Methodist Medical Center of Illinois with both hospitals providing academic support. We continued to lack formal structure and brand identification as a neurological destination center. In 1991, I talked with the administrators of both hospitals and the University of Illinois regarding the formation of the Illinois Neurological Institute, primarily to formalize the organization within the hospitals supporting the residency and provide a base for clinical research.

I hoped that over time, we might associate the name with significant clinical activity to form a successful Midwestern clinical care "brand". The Dean of the College of Medicine in Chicago advised me involvement with the University would result in a long delay. Founded primarily as a support mechanism for the University residency programs, the INI remained a hospital administrative structure, a cooperative educational venture of Saint Francis Medical Center and Methodist Medical Center. We designed a logo incorporating the state silhouette with a head and brain inside. This INI organization remained for nine years supporting the residency programs. Competitive forces made us unsuccessful in mounting joint INI clinical programs in both hospitals. Meanwhile, we continued to add faculty in neurology and neurosurgery in the clinical practice and subspecialty centers.

A bricks and mortar neurological institute dedicated to both the care of patients with illness of the nervous system and to understanding the diseases and the function of the nervous system remained my undeveloped vision. In spring 2001, wishing to create a hospital within a hospital like the Children's Hospital at Saint Francis Medical Center, and Barrow Neurological Institute at Saint Joseph Hospital, I talked with Mr. Keith Steffen, the President and CEO of Saint Francis Medical Center regarding formation of an Institute. Keith was supportive, and it was time to move ahead. The Illinois Neurological Institute would include neurology, neurosurgery, physical medicine and rehabilitation, neuro-radiology, neuropathology, and neurological radiation oncology. Saint Francis Medical Center closed the inpatient psychiatric unit several years before making it impossible to incorporate psychiatry.

I became the Director of the Illinois Neurological Institute (INI) at Saint Francis Medical Center that spring. Sue Wozniak, the COO of Saint Francis Medical Center, asked Deborah Richardson, Director of Outpatient Care, to assume the role of INI nursing director. Richardson later was named INI Vice President and Chief Operating Officer.

Our objective was a complete integration of the continuum of care from the first contact in the outpatient clinic, through hospital care, to rehabilitation and full recovery. Outpatient clinics were developed at a nearby building on Randolph Street for neurology and rehabilitation, and a specialty neurology center was built on the 6th floor of the hospital. Over time, the neurological intensive care and acute neurology floors were remodeled and developed, and a new intermediate care unit created. Richardson integrated the management of inpatient and outpatient units in a seamless process for patient care. To continue the development of the destination center, in 2008, OSF HealthCare System acquired the Associated Neurological Surgeons clinical practice.

In 2019, the INI is a 100-bed neurological institute within a large general hospital, with a neurological ICU, intermediate care unit, acute neurology floor and an inpatient rehabilitation floor. The Milestone Wing surgery unit contains two large general neurosurgery rooms, a two-room diagnostic-intraoperative MRI (iMRI) operating room, and the pediatric neurosurgery OR. A spinal surgery room is equipped with an O arm guidance system. A PerfeXion Gamma Knife and Varian TruBeam linear accelerator in radiation oncology support the INI Radiosurgery program. The INI Comprehensive Stroke Center utilizes two interventional neuroradiology rooms. The outpatient clinics on campus are located in a dedicated three-story clinic building adjacent to the inpatient service and the Jump Trading Simulation and Education Center.

Sixteen subspecialty centers are in varied states of development: Comprehensive Stroke Center, Spine Institute, Brain Tumor Center, Sleep Center, Comprehensive Level 4 Epilepsy Center, Neuro-ophthalmology Center, Balance and Vestibular Center, Multiple Sclerosis Center, Movement Disorders Center(Parkinson's Disease), Cognitive Disorders and Brain Health Center(Alzheimer's Disease), Neuro-muscular Center, Headache Center, and Pediatric Neuroscience Center. In addition to these centers, a Neurological Critical Care service and TeleNeurology program are in early development. An inpatient rehabilitation facility is integrated with multiple outpatient clinics providing convenient on-site rehabilitation. Some centers are fully developed and some remain in their infancy. The goal of each center is to provide the full spectrum of specialty care and a challenging residency and fellowship experience. Each multi-disciplinary specialty center is expected to create clinical and translational research programs to enhance clinical care, graduate education, and contribute to neurological knowledge.

In 1957, Penfield's vision of clinical medicine contributing new knowledge about the brain changed my life. In recent years, the development of clinical service lines and multiple competing centers make Penfield's and Bailey's approach to advancing science, while providing care, more difficult. Large integrated health systems may regard learning about how one thinks a dispensable luxury, to be accomplished by other centers. Research is integral to advancing modern medicine; clinicians fortunate enough to care for patients with complex neurological problems must contribute to the knowledge base of neuroscience.

An 80-Hour Work Week: Disruptive Change in Residencies

Training in the surgical specialties after finishing medical school in the '60s and '70s was a superhuman endurance contest. In some institutions, residents worked through the night several consecutive nights, and 100 hour work weeks were commonplace. The attending staff endured such a program, and they felt it was part of the initiation into the club. Functioning with sleep deprivation was a badge of honor. Over decades, a tradition of long hours, low pay, and minimal free time developed; all was felt to be an essential of "quality" residency training.

Libby Zion was seen in the emergency room, and died after admission to the New York Hospital in Manhattan in 1984. Review of her care raised concern; mistakes made in her care were the result of physician sleep deprivation. Concern regarding the safety of care provided by sleep-deprived residents escalated.

By 1989, New York State enacted regulations indicating residents could not work more than 80 hours per week, or more than 24 consecutive hours. This was a painful reduction for many famous academic surgical programs.

In July 2003, the Accreditation Council for Graduate Medical Education (ACGME), the residency accrediting body established national duty hour standards, and the hospital world changed dramatically. There was now an 80-hour weekly limit averaged over four weeks, with a ten hour rest period between duty periods and a 24 hour limit on continuous duty. New patients were not to be accepted after 24 hours of continuous duty. One day in seven was to be free of patient care and educational obligations. In house call could occur only every third night.

The new regulations reflected the findings of the rapidly developing field of sleep medicine demonstrating that sleep deprivation decreased efficiency and accuracy. There was a good deal of resistance to change in the leading neurosurgical programs. A limited number of 80-hour exceptions were granted for the chief resident. This exception allowed an 88-hour week, still a meaningful reduction. The change was in effect, was to be audited, and violation would result in loss of accreditation. Graduate training in the surgical specialties had undergone a disruptive change.

We immediately did a reassessment of the work done in the neurology and neurosurgery residency program, identifying elements critical to the educational process and service components that could be assumed by other members of the clinical team. I presented a request for an 88-hour week exemption for the chief resident in neurosurgery to the graduate education committee, mainly composed of internists and pediatricians. They denied the request, making it clear that the request was considered outrageous. A schism existed between the medical and surgical specialties; long hours were more ingrained in surgical training programs.

We committed to develop a group of advanced practice nurses and physician assistants trained in neurological care who would assume portions of the resident workload. Fortunately, neurosurgery had embarked on this course in a limited fashion earlier. Over the next 18 months, the residency program directors and Deborah Richardson, INI COO, developed a budget and recruitment program supporting the new residency work configuration. The INI soon had 20 APN's in place supporting the two services, assisting with the call schedule, and participating in patient care call responsibilities. We were in substantial compliance, with a less favorable cost structure.

The regulations were further modified, reducing the length of maximum service for interns or first-year residents to 16 hours. The issue continues to be studied by those responsible for graduate education. The work-hour solution has created new problems, while diminishing some of the problems associated with sleep deprivation. Frequent change of the physician responsible for patient care has increased the number of handoffs or transitions in the responsibility in the care of critically ill patients. Faculty members are concerned that a general loss of a sense of complete responsibility to the patient has occurred, replaced by a shift work mentality. Appropriately, the handoff process has been studied extensively. Protocols developed to make the transfer of care fail-safe are not yet consistently utilized. In 2017, some flexibility in the requirements was introduced, and further study is encouraging that modification will improve patient care and resident education and health.

Specialties that involve developing procedural expertise have found that residents are graduating with less experience, thus the length of residency programs continues to be evaluated. All neurosurgical residencies are now seven years in duration, and formal minimum procedure numbers have been published for the first time, in an attempt to mandate operative experience. The nature of surgical training is that many of the essential technical skills are learned in the senior residency or "chief" period, and the work hour reduction has diminished the opportunity to acquire great expertise. There have been a few papers that seem to demonstrate increased patient morbidity, correlated with the hours per week reduction.

Scandinavian and UK services have reduced their hours more than the US ACGME standards and seem to have worked through the process. There clearly is no going back, and the challenge is to use simulation and other techniques to enhance technical skill acquisition. Medicine historically has been somewhat slow to utilize technology in the improvement of training. Learning at the operating table, without adequate preliminary training and practice, is now unacceptable. Demonstrated competence in simulation will become a prerequisite for operating room opportunity.

The handoff transfer of care continues to require process improvement. With shorter hours and required days away, transfer of care is frequent. Recent studies in surgical residencies have demonstrated that introducing duty-hour flexibility, while maintaining the total hour requirements, did not alter the measures of safety or resident satisfaction significantly. (1, 2) Young physicians no longer expect to work inordinately long hours and our health care system will probably redesign the care model. It will require more physicians and teams of providers and will be more expensive until we redesign care processes. The most successful systems have a sense of urgency in this process.

Physical Medicine and Rehabilitation (PMR) in a Health Care System

Physical therapy and rehabilitation, when included in treatment planning from the onset of care, enhance recovery from disabling neurological illness. Rehabilitation planned and initiated before major elective surgical intervention facilitates rapid recovery. We included rehabilitation as a major element of the program at the formation of the Illinois Neurological Institute. Although this organization seemed rational, the physical therapy staff were initially uncomfortable being considered part of the Institute.

The staff wished to remain in their hospital administrative structure, and this change was unwelcome. Physical medicine and rehabilitation support many specialties, and multiple administrative structures are utilized in healthcare systems. There is a great deal of orthopedic illness requiring physical therapy. In the United States, private orthopedic groups provide physical therapy in their clinics, and that is true in the Peoria metropolitan area. An academic neuroscience referral center requires a broad spectrum of physical medicine and rehabilitation services in integrated multidisciplinary clinics. This was the fundamental reason for including PMR administratively in the Illinois Neurological Institute.

This was my first experience with poorly executed change. Our physical therapists and occupational therapists did not understand this "neurological designation". They did not feel they belonged in the INI. I had proceeded without consultation and staff participation. Because I knew where we were going, I assumed everyone understood where we were going; they did not. They had not participated in the planning. A significant blunder of business school proportion!

Deborah Richardson, a seasoned nurse administrator, immediately recognized the problem and set up multiple lunch meetings with small groups of the staff. We explained what was happening, the mission and commitment and their role, and fielded all questions. Change management required four months. A valuable lesson learned late. My previous life as a surgeon and a university "Professor and Head" simply had not developed my communication and people skills. Surgeons, historically, are noto-rious for a "Command" approach. Command does not work. Rapid remediation was sorely needed. The attitudes of my former life as a surgeon would not work while leading a neurological institute.

Just as in the other specialties of the Illinois Neurological Insti-tute, the rehabilitation program requires comprehensive, highly specialized destination programs serving patients with major and often rare problems. Geographically dispersed, readily available therapy services for the disabled incapable of extensive travel are also essential. Two very different strategies are required; one to treat rare complex problems in the center, one to address common problems with local convenience. When patients are in acute pain, they need to be seen that day with an initiation of treatment, rather than wait weeks for an appointment with a specialist. Major opportunities for improvement in access are achieved utilizing care pathways in musculoskeletal illness, supported by a well-developed system of outpatient therapy facilities. These facilities support the primary care practices in the acute and chronic management of many clinical problems.

When you cannot get out of bed after shoveling snow, an appoint-ment with a specialist in four weeks does not cut it, something better must be done. Dispersed outpatient physical therapists are a point of intake for acute neck and back pain. Well-developed care pathways allow early acute treatment with appropriate imaging and decreased invasive pain procedures. Extensive development of a back pain clinical pathway in Saskatchewan, Canada has demonstrated the utilization of physical therapists in the initial evaluation and care of acute spinal pain (1). Virginia Mason Spine Clinic in Seattle has incorporated physiatrists and physical thera-pists in a spine care clinic providing same-day access and prompt treatment.

Fall potential evaluation and therapeutic balance programs

offer an opportunity to better serve the aging population. Balance evaluation programs that are small and relatively inexpensive now make multiple geographically dispersed facilities feasible for patient convenience. As the patient mix in most health care systems evolves, with 25% of the patients 70 years or older, fall prevention is an essential priority in population health.

Driving competence assessment entails a more elaborate facility and is a destination function with an associated remediation and rehabilitation program for patients who are potential candidates for return to driving. This is an important element in the rehabilitation of stroke and brain injury patients.

Outpatient physical and occupational therapy support is involved in the destination comprehensive clinics in multiple sclerosis, movement disorders, neuromuscular disorders, stroke, and brain tumor. PMR space and facilities are incorporated in these clinics. Many of these patients come from a distance and are immobilized by their illness, making it critical that we go to them, rather than requiring their movement within a medical complex. When a multiple sclerosis patient is seen, the objective is to have the therapist go to the patient, rather than expect the patient to make a long trip to physical therapy.

A neurological institute needs either an integral inpatient rehabilitation unit, or a free-standing, nearby center in the same community. If an integral unit, a rapid transfer from acute care to rehabilitation is feasible, and early involvement in acute care is readily accomplished. A sub-specialized destination portfolio of services must reflect the population served by the health care system. Larger systems include a protective unit for young head injury patients, allowing a vigorous rehabilitation program without danger of patient elopement. It is a challenge to let young people with impaired judgment associated with head injury move about, allowing recovery without exposing them to further damage. Systems serving a large trauma catchment require a spinal cord injury program with appropriate orthotic service. A great deal of research in assistive robotics offers hope to these patients.

Physician staffing of dispersed outpatient clinics and specialized destination inpatient rehabilitation programs is challenging because of workforce shortages and the vagaries of funding and reimbursement. In recent years, the emphasis has been placed on EMG and pain management in physiatry training programs because both are well funded. This is an example of medical care dictated by reimbursement rather than population needs. EMG reimbursement was markedly reduced, and the value of epidural steroids and other injection methods are undergoing further investigation of their value. We are in the early stages of correction of reimbursement for patient value.

Timely physical therapy and rehabilitation programs have potential for reducing inappropriate imaging, reducing disability, and providing a rapid return to employment and full activity. The return on investment (ROI) continues to be a challenge in the design of programs. Decisions in this area are at the cutting edge of the transition from volume to value. To date, insurance plans have tended to compensate for MRI, epidural steroids, and have been less aggressive in paying for treatment resulting in prompt return to full activity and work. Often tests and procedures that do not add value are well compensated, and more simple effective care is not. (1) In a health system funded for value, models providing same day therapy will be financially and clinically sound.

A neurological institute preparing for the future needs to work with functional neurosurgery, in the area of cortical implants and robotic orthotics, to provide support for patients experiencing brain and spinal cord injury. These are active research areas requiring neurosurgical and physical medicine integration. Doctoral programs in physical therapy are adding staff prepared to enter research-oriented careers. Computer brain interfaces

214

driving prosthetic limbs and supportive devices will develop, becoming an integral part of rehabilitation programs. The Department of Defense continues substantial funding in support of these programs. Malcolm Gay describes this high tech race to merge minds and machines in his book *The Brain Electric*. (2)

Aneurysm Controlled:
All is Well, then Trouble

Sue Noble, a 38-year-old, right-handed secretary, came to the emergency room with a severe sudden headache in the late evening. She was alert, could speak and had no paralysis but did have a stiff neck. The "thunderclap" or sudden severe headache with the neck tightness was characteristic of subarachnoid hemorrhage (bleeding into the fluid around the brain) from an aneurysm. A CT scan revealed a good deal of blood in the subarachnoid space about the brain. Dr. Wright did angiography several hours later, revealing an 8mm aneurysm (25 mm=1 inch) at the carotid-posterior communicating artery junction on the left side, just after the carotid artery enters the skull cavity. This had leaked and the chances were very high that it would burst again soon causing death or extensive paralysis.

I performed surgery early the next morning making a scalp incision in back of the hairline, opening the skull at her temple. The base of the skull was drilled away, and the dura, the covering of the brain, opened. The cerebrospinal fluid was drained, the brain gently elevated and the carotid artery exposed next to the optic nerve at the base of the brain. A small balloon protruded from the carotid artery at the origin of the posterior communicating artery. The blood swirled in the thin-walled aneurysm. I placed a small 760 Yasargil clip across the base of the aneurysm then put a fine needle in the aneurysm, thus collapsing the sac. Opening the aneurysm assured that it was defused. After inspection to be sure that the clip closed no small arterial branches, the brain was allowed to settle back into position and the incision closed. Surgery had gone well and a little over two hours had passed.

Sue awakened promptly with a headache, and each day seemed more comfortable and alert. On the seventh day, Sunday morning, she mixed up a few words when I talked with her on my morning rounds at 7 am. She was experiencing vasospasm, the most dreaded and frequent complication after surgery for subarachnoid hemorrhage. The blood vessels clamp down, starving the brain's oxygenation, usually 7-10 days after the initial hemorrhage. This risk is generally proportional to the amount of initial bleeding, and Sue had had an extensive hemorrhage. I came back several hours later, before leaving the hospital. She now definitely had a right facial weakness, language difficulty, and a little weakness in her right arm and leg; she was clearly getting worse. I increased the IV fluids, returned her to the ICU, and gave drugs to elevate her blood pressure, with some improvement in her speech. In the next four days, constant changes in her speech and arm weakness were a source of recurring alarm. Angiography revealed profound spasm of the blood vessels in her brain, especially on the left side about the site of the aneurysm. We used all of the treatments available (triple therapy-elevate blood pressure-increase volume with IV fluids –hemodilution to increase blood flow). On the 14th day, she still had some language difficulties and moderate weakness in her right hand. Over a few months, with physical therapy, some further improvement occurred, but enough speech deficit and arm weakness remained to prevent return to her secretarial position. The course of her life was irreversibly altered, despite prompt treatment that seemingly had gone well. This was happening too often in patients with subarachnoid hemorrhage.

Causation of delayed cerebral ischemia, in essence, a stroke after subarachnoid hemorrhage, remained a mystery. The occurrence was only slightly predictable, and the treatment was unsatisfactory. This continuing problem led us to one of the first clinical research projects in our residency program.

Effective Treatment after Aneurysmal Rupture: Clinical Research

Mike Medlock completed medical school at the University of Florida and trained in pediatrics. He became interested in intensive care of children and took a fellowship in pediatric critical care at Baylor in Houston. This led to a decision to be a pediatric neurosurgeon, and that brought him to Peoria in 1988. Mike finished the program at the INI in 1994 and went to a pediatric neurosurgery fellowship at Boston Children's Hospital, Harvard Medical School. He later joined the staff at the Massachusetts General Hospital in Boston.

Mike, while the chief resident, was interested in critical care aspects of subarachnoid hemorrhage and clinical research. We decided to manage our subarachnoid hemorrhage patients with a standard treatment protocol to decrease the risk of stroke caused by vasospasm. Blood volume expansion (increasing the amount of circulating blood) would be employed to improve the cerebral circulation.

We placed tubing (Swan-Ganz catheter) through the right side of the heart into the pulmonary artery that carried blood to the lungs. Intravenous fluid was administered as tolerated to increase heart output, thus improving blood flow to the brain. If fluid administration were overdone, fluid accumulated in the lungs producing what is termed pulmonary edema with heart failure. We hoped to avoid pulmonary edema by monitoring pressure in the pulmonary artery via the catheter. We treated 146 patients for subarachnoid hemorrhage during the study period, and 61 patients satisfied the requirements of the study design. Pulmonary edema occurred in 12 patients and infection related to the catheter in 3 patients required prolonged antibiotic management.

We showed that preventive aggressive blood volume expansion was associated with significant complications. Efficacy in preventing delayed ischemia or stroke with this addition to conventional management was not demonstrated. Although a randomized controlled trial would have been more conclusive, our study was frequently quoted as demonstrating the problems associated with prophylactic hypervolemia management. This problem continues to be studied in many centers with limited incremental improvement.

In recent years, we have utilized physical dilation of the artery in spasm with an intra-arterial catheter and balloon and drug therapy introduced in the artery. Post hemorrhage vasospasm continues to be an unpredictable problem in the care of severe subarachnoid hemorrhage and still lacks an entirely effective treatment. Delayed cerebral ischemia remains a black cloud over aneurysm care.

Electronic Medical Record: Progress, not a Panacea

After a great deal of study, comparison and analysis, OSF Health-Care System decided on EPIC as an electronic medical record. The old handwritten medical record had many defects, and pressure was building to use computer data systems to fix the deficiencies in medical records. OSF HealthCare elected to change all elements of the record in a single step at each of their facilities, rather than a piecemeal adoption. The old handwritten paper record would disappear overnight.

EPIC is a company in Verona, Wisconsin, near Madison, that

began developing a system to manage the business aspects of clinical practice. Over time, the company product gradually evolved to offer a complete clinical record. When OSF HealthCare selected this system, EPIC was one of the three leading providers of electronic health records in the United States. OSF had used IDX, a system generated by a firm in Vermont, acquired by General Electric. General Electric failed to create an enduring solution, and transition to a system that would meet future needs was required.

The primary care practices of the OSF HealthCare Medical Group first implemented EPIC in 2008. We planned to take each hospital "live" sequentially, implementing the entire program in one step at each facility, termed the "Big Bang Approach". Virtually all of the employees had some relationship to the medical record, creating a monumental educational challenge. Medical staff, nursing staff, and various therapy and technical staff members, all had unique educational needs. The time available was limited with tight deadlines. A commitment to the process evolved as everyone participated in the required classroom and individual remediation. A few physicians and nurses near retirement elected to leave, unwilling to deal with the electronic health record and computers.

Adapting to EPIC was a painful process; hours of instruction by young people who were very computer literate, very familiar with the software, but did not seem to entirely understand the objective in the medical record. I persisted because there was no alternative, and I believed that ultimately we would improve care. A difficult transition for an experienced surgeon accustomed to performing competently; it reminded me of my attempts at watercolor. The worst painter in the class.

The individual hospitals were phased in over a year, beginning with OSF Saint Anthony Medical Center, Rockford in December 2009. Saint Anthony, with 220 beds, was large enough to adequately test the system and learn a great deal, but posed a limited risk for clinical function and cash flow because it was not the largest facility. The early months were painful. Services were not billed, and the cash flow at SAMC was seriously impacted. The choice to go live in the smaller facility was validated, the process tested, and although cash flow was impaired for several months, it was tolerable. Virtually all of the medical staff actively participated in the process, a critical element in the success at SAMC.

Over 18 months, the remaining hospitals and outpatient practices installed EPIC, achieving a single medical record across OSF HealthCare System. The Illinois Neurological Institute outpatient clinics went live on November 16, 2012. In the ensuing several years, as national Medicare policy and private carrier contracts included expectations for electronic medical record compliance and meaningful usage, it was clear the decision to proceed, and the overall timing and execution were excellent. EPIC serves many large medical centers, with the largest market share (approximately 20% of the national market and a significantly larger percentage of academic medical centers).

Ten years after implementation, it is possible to make some observations. Marked differences of opinion exist in this matter, but the positive effects are:

1. The medical record is legible; handwriting errors are eliminated.

2. The medical record is immediately widely available throughout the healthcare system, saving time in transmission of records, filing, mailing etc., and avoiding delays in care because of the lack of records.

3. Medication reconciliation (Preparation of an accurate list of the patient's medications at each point in the process of care) has resulted in significant reduction in medication errors, and electronic prescriptions have reduced error.

4. Some improvement in care processes has occurred with advice and hard stops incorporated in the EPIC process. The record system can make it challenging to create orders inappropriate to the patient's condition. Hard stops, in some cases, make it impossible to proceed without clarification of an issue in question.

There are disappointments associated with the process and opportunities exist:

1. There are at least 15 vendors with some share in the market. From the beginning, neither the government nor the industry developed requirements for compatibility in record systems that addressed the nation's need for a national system of healthcare. Each EPIC installation is different in some aspects so that even EPIC installations do not interact seamlessly, although this challenge is being addressed. As the federal government required and financially supported a transition to the electronic record, it missed an opportunity to implement compatibility requirements. This was a significant lost opportunity.

2. The quality of the medical record in some respects is worse. Care providers do a great deal of cutting and pasting, and succinct analysis is rare. Although supported by the software, this reflects shortcuts developed by physicians and providers. Physicians and nurses must place information in categorical segments allowing retrieval. This discourages free text with associated succinct, thoughtful analysis previously seen in the medical record. The computer fills in areas in the record with repetitive data making it difficult to find critical elements.

3. Billing requirements lead to onerous repetitious statements in physician and nursing notes, diminishing the

quality of the clinical record. Critical clinical data is sometimes obscured in the medical record by routine data supporting billing. This is not a direct effect of the electronic record, but the billing requirements of insurance companies and Medicare.

4. The Illinois Neurological Institute and OSF Neuroscience Service Line have yet to utilize the software to provide system-wide care pathways drastically improving patient care and safety. The potential for care improvement is slowed by the difficulty in effecting software change.

5. Data retrieval for clinical research and/or outcomes analysis entails laborious manual extraction processes. Some EPIC systems lack clinical research support. This need is acknowledged and work is in progress. Natural language processing is not utilized to extract information from free text.

6. Although some physicians have utilized the computer in a fashion avoiding intrusion in the patient relationship, others are viewed as more interested in their computer and record keeping than listening to the patient or teaching residents and medical students.

7. It is often difficult to order x-rays and medications. The software is viewed as "clunky and clumsy". Business and entertainment applications appear more intuitive than those provided for medical applications.

EPIC and other electronic health records are here to stay, and the potential for improving care processes is immense. Ultimately, it will become difficult to order an inappropriate test when seeing a seizure or brain tumor patient, and care pathways incorporated in the EPIC system will guide treatment. The challenge is to fully utilize the available computer and data power in the daily decision process. Execution requires young clinicians who have few convictions as to the "best way" to do things.

Introduction of the electronic health record has a significant economic impact on health systems. Cost of the software, extensive education cost and problems in coding and billing have invariably adversely affected budgets. In late 2015, the Brigham and Women's Hospital, a 793-bed hospital in Boston, part of the multi-hospital Partners HealthCare System, reported a $53 million shortfall caused by cost overruns in an EPIC implementation. Partners as a system budgeted $1.2 billion for EPIC installation.

Robert Wachter in his book *Digital Doctor: Hope, Hype, and Harm at the Dawn of Medicine's Computer Age* reviews the problems associated with excessive "cut and paste" and the voluminous redundant medical records created. (1) He relates in depth a patient who received 38 times the proper dose of Septra at UCSF hospital. Many mistakes were made, and some were related to the EHR. Wachter expresses the hope that with voice recognition, machine learning, artificial intelligence and natural language processing, the computers will be integrated into medical care with substantive benefits. His book discusses the detrimental effects of the EHR on clinical practice and potential benefits and future opportunities. Too many clicks are needed and it may be worse with ICD 10, the new coding system implemented nation-wide in October 2015. In most records, a succinct synopsis is lacking. Cut and paste is the anti-thesis of a thoughtful concise record. A hard stop requiring a fresh analysis of the problem daily would be a programming challenge but an invaluable improvement. Unlimited opportunities for improvement remain. I am confident that the electronic health record will ultimately realize it's potential for improving American health care.

Part II

Meeting the Twenty-First Century Challenge in Neuroscience

Chapter 8

INI and OSF
Neuroscience Service Line
2008-2014

A physician is obligated to consider more than
a diseased organ, more than the whole man —
he must view the man in his world

—Harvey Cushing

INI and OSF
Neuroscience Service Line

In 2008, OSF HealthCare created the OSF Neuroscience Service Line to provide neurological care for the population served by the multi-hospital system. Hospital systems were creating service lines to achieve efficiency, quality, and marketing goals. Service line leadership of neurological care in the multi-hospital system was a dramatic change in OSF HealthCare strategy. OSF functioned as a holding company model with substantial independence for each operating unit. Nationally, most large hospital systems were performing as holding companies, and the concept of system service line was in its infancy. At inception, we did not realize the culture change required to achieve an operating company. This service line was to be more than a marketing function; it was to provide the same care to patients regardless of point of entry in the system. We underestimated the complexity of the challenge.

After a limited internal search in October 2008, I became the CEO of the INI and the OSF Neuroscience Service Line. I planned to develop the Illinois Neurological Institute (INI) in Peoria as a destination neurological center supporting specialized neurological care for the population served by OSF HealthCare System. We needed to determine what care could be provided in each local facility, avoiding unproductive patient and family travel. Optimum quality and value of neuroscience care in all of OSF HealthCare System was our commitment. We began the creation of an integrated system with similar care paths, metrics, and quality of care regardless of point of entry in the system. A remarkably simple concept that proved difficult to execute.

OSF HealthCare provides neurological care in Peoria, Rockford, Alton, Bloomington, Urbana, Danville, and a number of smaller Illinois communities. These services lacked a defined relationship with the INI in Peoria. The challenge was to build a system-wide program that served the neurological needs of the entire population.

Population health is currently thought to involve primary care, preventive medicine, and public health. Neuroscience is responsible for the care of many people with stroke, trauma, sleep disorders, epilepsy, dementia, and other degenerative disorders of increasing importance as the population ages. Virtually all of our physicians considered their patients those that presented for care, rather than all in the general population inadequately served or diagnosed. Acceptance of a population responsibility shared with all of the providers within the OSF HealthCare System represented a substantial change. As a group, those unseen patients had not been their responsibility. Acceptance of responsibility for "patients not yet seen" is critical to the long-term care of large populations. This fundamental change in attitude has not occurred in specialty medicine.

Primary care leadership accepted the population health concept intellectually, but were not executing improvement in population care. Specialty medicine did not recognize the problem. A ten-week waiting list was a matter of pride; an indication of superiority, "everyone wants to see me." Specialists do not acknowledge their role in an unseen patient going blind with papilledema while awaiting an initial appointment. Lack of a timely appointment is their responsibility just as much as the patient sitting across from them in the office. That was the situation in 2008, and remains the problem a decade later with little apparent progress.

The Illinois Neurological Institute and the OSF Neuroscience Service Line are two different related and supportive entities. The INI continues to develop a specialty destination referral center providing OSF HealthCare and other healthcare systems high quality specialized, research supported centers unavailable in their facility. The INI offers a specialty care solution to other health care systems and smaller centers within OSF HealthCare, unable to provide complex low volume care. Some centers in the INI, to thoroughly develop their clinical, educational, and research mission require a large population base only achieved with relationships with other health care systems with different strengths. The INI offers a solution to portfolio deficiencies as a specialty center growth strategy.

The OSF Neuroscience Service Line is responsible for delivering neuroscience population health to those we serve. This role involves a different strategy than the destination center. Integration with primary care and other departments and centers within OSF, to make the whole more effective than the sum of the parts, is the guiding principle of the service line. In October 2008, each of the 16 INI Specialty Centers was charged with responsibility for care across OSF Health Care. In 2019, this includes 14 hospitals serving a broad geography. At the outset, neither the individual specialty groups nor the disparate operating units understood the implications of this charge, or the complexity of execution. It has been a challenging period, and perhaps a third of the objective has been met. In the next few pages, I will review the role of these centers in future health care. The methods and strategies to execute population health responsibilities in a destination center are addressed.

The fall of 2008, as INI embarked on this program, the United States entered the most severe financial crisis experienced since the great depression. Freezing of credit markets in October 2008 added to the complexity of execution. During this period of capital immobilization in the United States, time was lost in implementation. The experience demonstrated that a sound strategy is not determined quarterly. We made small adjustments, while remaining focused on the long-term need.

Advice Needed:
The INI Advisory Board is Created

The INI at OSF Saint Francis Medical Center developed as a destination referral neuroscience center from 2001; the creation of the OSF Neuroscience Service Line in 2008, added new challenges and responsibilities. I was concerned we were insular doctors talking to other doctors and nurses and lacked the voice of the community and insight of industry, outside of health care. Some non-healthcare sectors were rapidly solving problems with data management and technology. We needed to capture their experience and fresh ideas.

I asked our CEO, Mr. James Moore, if I might develop an INI Advisory Board. He agreed an advisory board would offer value and brought the proposal to the OSF Governing Board, who gave approval to proceed. After seeking advice from many sources, I asked Gerry Shaheen to chair the new advisory board over breakfast oatmeal at our local Bob Evans restaurant. Gerry questioned me at length; he had an interest in improving healthcare with process and data management. At the time, Mr. Shaheen was Chairman of the Board of Bradley University, and a board member of Ford and Agro, a large farm machinery company. Gerry had recently retired as Group President for mining and construction equipment at Caterpillar and had a full schedule. He did not wish to commit unless he could contribute and promised a decision in 30 days.

Gerry called three weeks later; he would help create an INI board. We met again, discussed the board size and he proposed additional members. Extensive board experience led Gerry to suggest a small, intensely involved group. I had initially envisioned 12-15 members. Gerry advised a group half that size; small groups were responsible, not observers. In the next month, he and

I had breakfast with each prospective member, discussing the INI, it's mission, and work to be accomplished.

Larry Wallden, former group president of Caterpillar Asia, brought a strong background in sales. He had worked in Africa, Switzerland, and multiple locations in Asia. Larry was a man who didn't take "no" for an answer, and was committed to making a difference. He had received a diagnosis of Multiple Sclerosis when near retirement and was determined that the INI would offer the best MS center possible. He already had provided critical guidance as we developed a strategic plan for Multiple Sclerosis.

The next breakfast brought on board Ed Rapp, Caterpillar Chief Financial Officer. Ed brought formidable financial, planning, and execution skills. Mr. Rapp was from a small town in Missouri and understood the needs of those we serve. Responsible for legal and financial divisions, he had acquired expertise in the recruitment of skilled professionals to small town mid-America, a critical problem for the INI.

Jonathan Michael, CEO of RLI, an international insurance firm, provided experience with risk management and the insurance industry. Jonathan was a thoughtful listener who built consensus. He reminded INI leadership to involve users when creating solutions. Jonathan demonstrated a commitment to team involvement. He brought inherent optimism and a "can do" spirit to discussions. RLI was founded in Peoria by Gerald Stephens to provide insurance to replace contact lenses. The company broadened its role over the years and remained committed to Peoria. RLI has an ownership relationship with Maui Jim sunglasses, also in Peoria. At a board meeting, with a smile, he put on distinctive orange reading glasses to peruse a document. An upbeat original member with a sense of humor.

Jim Cote, CEO of Sanders Tool, brought skills in operations and management. Jim, a big athletic man, was a man of action interested in practical details of providing excellent service to our patients. Mr. Cote always reminded me of the operational details so critical to execution.

I asked Dr. Walter Whisler from Chicago to join the board. Walt was an old friend and Emeritus Professor and Chairman of Neurosurgery at Rush University. Dr. Whisler provided insight regarding relationship management in large hospitals that he acquired while serving many years in one of the largest systems in the Chicago area. He contributed knowledge of the Chicago and Northern Illinois market and his experience with multiple large health care systems. Walt's extensive experience in developing academic research programs spoke to one of the INI's pressing needs.

The board met every 60 days for 2 hours with a well-planned agenda and background material provided in advance. Mr. Shaheen had managed meetings his entire career and brought direction and structure to the board. The members received the agenda and a "board book" of background material 10 days before each meeting. We started on time, ended on time, stayed on focus, and made decisions. Digression did not occur. The board acted as consultants for problems in execution and strategy. Their insight on customer service and marketing was invaluable. The small size of the board made each member a vigorous participant, rather than an observer. If a member was away from the city, they made arrangements to call in or "Skype". Their commitment to our success was wondrous and sustained. Their respect for one another and their complementary expertise fostered intense discussion. Each meeting closed with a brief meeting of the board with me after other participants were excused. Invaluable advice from "my consultants". Their support and enthusiasm was palpable, a treasured experience.

A number of the INI Advisory Board sessions were memorable. Ed Rapp talked with us regarding setting the cadence of a project. He discussed developing a new program, with intermediate deadlines, and meetings to evaluate progress. It seemed that generally in health care, we had a meeting, and then had another in 1-3 months, sometimes to find that little had transpired in the interim. In Ed's meetings with his direct reports, the cadence was much faster; the next meeting in one week with clear achievement expectations. We were viewing execution in a fast moving, highly competitive industry with precise metrics; the future state for medical care. Ed Rapp introduced the concept and considered at length the significant culture change required to make it happen in healthcare.

A recurring challenge was the INI brand and its role in OSF HealthCare and Saint Francis Medical Center. Although Saint Francis was the fourth largest hospital in Illinois, OSF HealthCare was a medium sized, multiple hospital system. The INI had a number of specialty services, such as the INI Brain Tumor Center and Neuro-Ophthalmology, requiring a large population base. We needed many referrals from other healthcare systems to achieve ambitious goals; we were to be a portfolio solution for other systems. Although the INI is wholly owned by OSF HealthCare, it gradually developed a distinct reputation and brand value. The INI Advisory Board members contributed their extensive experience to our brand deliberations and development.

Brand strategy in healthcare continues to evolve and become more complex. Health systems are becoming larger, more comprehensive, and less tolerant of out-migration. I believe there will continue to be opportunities as portfolio design is driven by increasingly stringent economic constraints. Outsourcing by smaller health systems of some complex specialty care to destination centers will be a sound strategy for all parties. The niche markets will influence brand strategy.

Changes in Caterpillar's Asia market required Mr. Rapp's transfer to Singapore, and Mr. Seshadri Guha replaced him on the INI Advisory Board. Guha founded GGN Global, a consulting firm in

Peoria with a worldwide practice that was developing an interest in medical process improvement. Guha added to the Board a great deal of expertise in process analysis.

The same year, Dr. Gerald McShane, the president of the OSF Medical Group joined the board, providing assurance INI remains aware of its role and responsibility to the entire OSF population. Gerry brought Medical Group service concerns to our attention immediately.

The major contribution of the Board with Mr. Shaheen's leadership was to probe and remove us from the insular mindset of the medical industry. The board made us aware of non-medical industry methods to attack problems and constantly reminded us of what people want. A weekly review of published hospital administration journals suggests that groupthink exists in healthcare, and the insight of other industries is invaluable. This small highly involved board bimonthly pulled us out of the world of healthcare and made us confront our responsibility to society. The board's well-prepared respectful debate and analysis set a standard for the self-satisfied providers of healthcare.

Integrated Care at the INI:
Population Health in Neuroscience

The sections of this chapter consider the challenges associated with caring for a large Midwestern population with neurological illness; our experience at the Illinois Neurological Institute, and future challenges and opportunities. The INI was organized with sixteen specialty centers responsible for the health of the population served. Our goal at onset was an integrated system, avoiding the creation of islands. Although each specialty center was unique, a common vision, commitment, and responsibility was expected.

Clinical care is provided by a team of physicians, APN's, nurses, neuropsychologists, therapists, social workers and ancillary staff, each possessing expertise in their specialty. They develop care processes and support the work of the health care system. Each center is addressing the need to provide both central specialized services and dispersed services required by complex disabling neurological illness. Supportive care is provided to patients and families dealing with the unique stresses generated by neurological illness.

Centers participate in nursing, medical student, resident, and continuing education programs. Programs utilizing technology and simulation are in active development by a few of the specialty centers. Some of the specialty centers have yet to fully address the opportunities offered by technology and simulation.

Centers are expected to develop clinical research and some have basic science and translational programs as well. Each will develop databases supporting process improvement and clinical research.

Brain Tumor

Viewed from the perspective of population health, brain tumor occurs infrequently. When it involves your family, it immediately becomes one of life's worst and most important events. Caring for brain tumor patients and their families has been challenging and rewarding; yet at times with failure, heartbreaking. Presenting infrequently in the practice of those in general medicine, brain tumor diagnosis is often delayed and initial treatment sub-optimal, adding to the pain suffered by patients and families.

Unfortunately, brain tumors are not as uncommon as thought by primary care physicians. A brain tumor brings fear and sadness to many patients and families. Brain tumor is the second leading cause of cancer-related death in children under 20 (1st cause is leukemia), the second leading cause of cancer-related death in males 20-39(1st cause is leukemia) and the fifth leading cause in females aged 20-39. Gliomas (tumors arising in the supporting structure of the brain) represent 30% of brain tumors. The most malignant of the gliomas, glioblastoma, represents 17% of primary brain tumors. The prevalence rate of brain tumor is 221.8 per 100,000 persons with about 69,000 new tumors, 24,000 malignant and 45,000 non-malignant diagnosed per year in the United States. (1)

Metastatic tumors, tumors that have spread from primary cancers elsewhere in the body, are the most common brain tumor. Although the national metastatic data is not as accurate as primary tumor data, metastatic tumors are more common than primary tumors. Treatment of metastatic tumors has become necessary as improvement in systemic cancer treatment results in patients living a longer life. For some patients, cancer is now a chronic disease requiring years of recurring treatment. Technology and drug development steadily lead to improved complex care, providing advanced management of metastatic brain tumor.

A population base with numerous patients is essential for the full development of a multi-disciplinary comprehensive brain tumor center. The program must address the diagnosis, surgical care, radiation treatment, chemotherapy, rehabilitation, and supportive care for patients and families. Portions of this care are best provided in a central referral center, and a portion of the care can and should be provided near home in a dispersed arrangement.

Initial diagnosis is challenging because patients have diverse presenting symptoms. The region of the brain involved generates local symptoms, and general symptoms are caused by increased intracranial pressure. Initial diagnosis is often delayed by the general perception of rarity of brain tumor; the diagnosis is simply not considered. In the future, clinical decision software may aid prompt initial recognition and diagnosis by primary care physicians. Imaging with enhanced MRI is usually the definitive diagnostic test. Thirty years after the introduction of MRI, patients often still have a CT scan as their initial test for brain tumor, a wasteful unnecessary step. Failure of an inappropriate, less sensitive CT scan to reveal the tumor can delay diagnosis for months.

When initial images reveal a brain tumor, the remainder of the MRI sequences are optimally selected by an experienced brain tumor neuro-radiologist, decreasing the need for repeated additional scans yielding the information required for management decisions. The goal is each test provides maximum information, decreasing repetitive testing. Each tumor location and type has an optimal set of images to plan the operation or the next treatment step. Pituitary tumors require thin sections delineating the tumor and relationships to the optic nerves. Tumors in the language function filled dominant hemisphere require white matter fiber tract imaging for surgical planning.

System-wide Picture Archiving and Communication Systems (PACS) store X-ray, CT, and MRI images and make digital images available everywhere in the OSF HealthCare System regardless of location. PACS facilitates coordination of diagnosis and treatment planning by experienced radiologists. Achievement of the imaging goal requires recognition of information during initial sequences with customization of the subsequent imaging to provide required information. This entails major process and culture change in radiology departments. The patient currently receives a standard ordered image set, regardless of the result of early images. Process change will decrease cost, patient pain and suffering, and lost time. Tailoring of the study while in process is another illustration of precision medicine yet to be implemented. Decision support computer software with artificial intelligence (AI) will aid this process. When an abnormality is seen in early images, AI software could suggest an alteration in image selection.

We continue to work toward this goal in the INI, developing

care pathways in decision support software. It must first be accomplished in one hospital, then implemented across the system. Change in initial imaging tests requires a significant culture change in radiology systems; no radiology department can remain an island. PACS permits application of expertise generated anywhere in the system, and this value of PACS has not been widely utilized. Cost containment will inevitably drive change currently impeded by a tradition of independent radiology departments.

Preoperative imaging provides information regarding brain function and fiber tract connection relationships; essentially a tumor treatment road map. When loaded into surgery guidance systems, safe complete tumor resection is accomplished with less postoperative neurological damage. At the current state of development, this necessitates qualified neuroradiology and MRI physics capability in the brain tumor center. New computer software permits evaluation of the extent of tumor removal as surgery is performed. Planning allows accurate intra-operative decisions regarding the optimum extent of tumor removal. Knowing when to stop during surgery avoids loss of neurological function. The potential of postsurgical radiosurgery treatment can be evaluated during the operation. In vestibular tumor removal from the seventh nerve (facial movement), a decision to leave a small piece of tumor in place to be treated with Gamma Knife radiosurgery decreases the risk of permanent facial paralysis caused by the the removal of a final small tumor section.

Intraoperative MRI imaging systems(over 60 in the United States) are now widely available in brain tumor centers permitting assessment of the adequacy of tumor removal before closure of the surgical incision. The INI brain tumor center has utilized intraoperative MRI since January 2016. To date, intraoperative MRI has had the greatest value in the surgery of low-grade glioma, skull base benign tumors and pituitary tumors. Imaging before completion of surgery assures the operative objective is achieved before the patient leaves the operating room. Patients harboring these tumors have the potential for long life with appropriate management. Intraoperative MRI suites are now also utilized for some less invasive treatments including laser treatment of deep small tumors and seizure foci.

A multidisciplinary brain tumor center requires a substantial physician team and staff. The INI recruited a neurosurgeon with neurosurgical oncology training committed to clinical care, education, and research who spends full time on the tumor program. Recent studies suggest that surgeons dedicated to brain tumor treatment achieve better results with lower cost. (2) Chemotherapy for brain tumor patients and expertise in paraneoplastic neurological syndromes associated with cancer is also provided by our neuro-oncologist. Three radiation oncologists, skilled in radiosurgery utilizing Gamma Knife and Linac, are critical to the INI brain tumor program. Treatment planning is supported by two physicists with extensive radiosurgery experience.

Endoscopy and temporal bone skull base techniques required in some pituitary and skull base tumors are contributed by an ear, nose, and throat (ENT) surgeon. A plastic surgeon with extensive craniofacial surgical experience is essential in a number of complex skull base tumor problems. The hormonal management of pituitary and para-sellar tumors is performed by a neuro-endocrinologist. Neuro-ophthalmology contributes to the evaluation of pituitary and para-sellar tumors as well as tumors affecting the extra-ocular movements and the visual pathways. A physiatrist with tumor experience provides expertise in rehabilitation, assuring optimum recovery. This multidisciplinary team provides the entire spectrum of evaluation, complex image- guided surgery, chemotherapy, and a complete radiation oncology program leading to maximum rehabilitation and function.

The neuropathologist is a critical member of the brain tumor team. Although the pathologist is essential in the study of the microscopic appearance of the tumor, patients with microscopically identical tumors sometimes have very different outcomes, particularly in patients with astrocytoma and oligodendroglioma. Genetic characteristics differentiate these tumors. Identifying patients' genetic and molecular characteristics is introducing "personalized medicine" to brain tumor care. The ability to identify and treat specific genetic molecular abnormalities provides hope that we will ultimately successfully treat a malignant brain tumor.

In gliomas of adult life, three molecular markers have undergone extensive studies in recent years: 1p/19q chromosomal codeletion, (6)-methylguanine methyltransferase (MGMT) promoter methylation, and mutations of isocitrate dehydrogenase (IDH) 1 and 2. In 2012, long-term follow-up of the Radiation Therapy Oncology Group Trial 9402 and the European Organization for Research and Treatment of Cancer Trial 26951 demonstrated an overall survival benefit from the addition of chemotherapy with procarbazine/CCNU/vincristine confined to patients with anaplastic oligodendroglial tumors with (vs. without) 1p/19q codeletion. This was a fundamental change; we could determine a patient group that could expect improvement with a specific new treatment.

In elderly glioblastoma patients, the NOA-08 and the Nordic randomized, phase 3 trial of radiation therapy (RT) alone versus temozolomide alone demonstrated a profound impact of MGMT promoter methylation on the outcome by therapy and, thus established MGMT as a predictive biomarker in this patient population. Thus, recent identification of the 1p/19q co-delation, and EDH, and TERT promoter mutations are more accurate identifiers than histology and probably eliminates mistakes associated with sample selection error. (4,5). Previously, a sampling error could be introduced by selecting a more non-malignant section of the tumor for biopsy. Although this is complex, it simply shows that analysis of the genetic makeup of a tumor allows better prediction of response to treatment than previously used microscopic diagnosis. These changes are reflected in the 2016 World Health Organization Classification of tumors of the central nervous system which relates to the phenotype and genotype of the tumor. (6)

These studies illustrate the precision management attainable in brain tumor care. (4) The risk of enduring side effects from a medication or ineffective treatment is diminished by tumor genotyping. This is the cutting edge of "precision medicine". Patients do better if they receive precise treatment and avoid treatments that do not have value. Time is not lost and the associated side effects are minimized. Progress in glioma brain tumor management often means extending the patient's life by several months; a truly disruptive breakthrough is still not apparent.

The infrastructure for a full clinical trial and clinical research program is necessary to recruit and retain a skilled team. The best people in the field want to understand better and improve brain tumor treatment. Patients with unsolved problems want to participate in clinical trials that offer hope. The tumor database optimally should be incorporated as an integral part of the health care system electronic health record, supporting continuous analysis of quality and a publication program, as well. The INI has yet to achieve this degree of operational management utilizing EPIC; it remains an elusive goal.

A brain tumor center must be financially self-sustaining over time. If this described extensive facility is utilized at capacity, the brain tumor Disease Related Group (DRG) provides a significant contribution margin. The optimum center function requires 200+ new tumors per year, with 40 high-grade gliomas diagnosed per year, and a program for management of metastatic brain disease at optimum level. The INI brain tumor sees over 300 new brain tumor patients each year. In a multiple hospital system, this necessitates designation of a single specialty center with a commitment to utilization of specialty facilities. Health care systems were assembled from previously free-standing units in a holding system retaining autonomy. Most have yet to achieve the integration of an operating system. Integration entails change in clinical behavior, disrupting referral patterns. An earlier culture with neurosurgeons doing 6-8 brain tumor operations per year is incompatible with current technology and quality transparency.

The highly technical aspects of surgical and radiation care must be performed in a high volume center. A healthcare system serving extensive geography provides follow up and support mechanisms close to home in regional centers eliminating unnecessary travel for patients and family. Physiotherapy, supportive counseling, chemotherapy, and fractionated radiation may be provided away from the destination center, using system care plans for guidance. The distant follow-up care is a continuum with the initial care. Data accumulated in the system-wide tumor database supports optimum care and continuous evaluation of long term program quality.

The INI Brain Tumor board meets weekly to review patients utilizing the expertise of all disciplines involved. Smart boards and PACS permit incorporation of consultation with distant hospitals in the system. To date, the technology is available, but we have yet to fully achieve consistent utilization of the health systems expertise. System-wide expertise must ultimately be applied to the care of each brain tumor patient. A work in progress requiring consistent system wide commitment.

Stroke Stopped

Ralph Black complained to his wife, Emma, that he just did not feel right around 3:30 on Saturday afternoon and decided to lie down on the couch. Ralph was a 47-year-old African American with a history of hypertension who smoked a pack of cigarettes a day but felt he was in good health, working each day on construction. At 5:00, while talking to Emma, his speech became garbled and he seemed to be looking away, and after several minutes stopped talking. He attempted to get up, and could not, his right arm and leg would not move. Emma called 911, and the ambulance arrived at 5:30. The Emergency Medical Service (EMS) technician detected the right-sided paralysis, loss of speech, and ignoral of the right side, indicating a probable large left-sided stroke. His NIH Stroke Scale was 24 (0 no stroke symptoms, 21-42 severe stroke). He was taken to the CT scan immediately. Imaging revealed no evidence of bleeding and the middle cerebral artery, the major artery to the central portion of the left brain was dense, suggesting a clot in the middle cerebral artery. tPA was administered immediately at 6:00 PM, one hour after stroke onset. The CT angiogram revealed occlusion of the main trunk of the middle cerebral artery, which is usually not cleared with IV treatment. The stroke neurologist arranged for Ralph to be taken immediately to the neurointerventional suite. Dr. Fraser, the neurointerventional radiologist, placed a needle in the femoral artery in the groin, introduced a catheter and did an angiogram demonstrating complete occlusion of the left middle cerebral artery. He removed the clot with suction, re-establishing blood flow to the central portion of the left side of Ralph's brain. Three and one-half hours had passed when Ralph returned to the intensive care unit. During the night, he regained motion in the arm and leg, and gradually began to understand and speak several words. After several days of further care and physical therapy, he returned home. When seen in the clinic three weeks later, his strength was normal and his speech and comprehension were minimally impaired. At this point, he had not returned to his work, but was fishing and playing softball. A life-changing disaster had been averted with a new approach to stroke.

In earlier years, we would have watched helplessly while Ralph developed loss of brain function. Instead of returning to an active life, Ralph would have joined the permanently disabled, perhaps consigned to a prolonged nursing home stay.

Cerebrovascular Illness and Stroke

Research in cerebrovascular disease and stroke care is a major commitment of neurology departments in the United States after years of therapeutic nihilism. Stroke continues to be a major population health problem. Although people fear stroke, their knowledge remains inadequate. In a 2005 survey, only 38% of the population was aware of significant stroke symptoms and knew to call 9-1-1 when someone is having a stroke (10). Stroke remains the fourth leading cause of death in the US and the leading cause of serious long-term disability with about 800,000 strokes per year in the United States costing an estimated $36.5 billion in health care services, medications, and missed work. Stroke is among the top 15 most expensive conditions treated in US Hospitals and among the top 10 most expensive conditions billed to Medicare. On a positive note, the incidence of stroke is falling, with a decrease of 14% in stroke deaths from 1995 to 2005. Improved management of atherosclerosis, hypertension, atrial fibrillation, and decreased smoking have all contributed to the gradual improvement.

A landmark paper in the *New England Journal of Medicine* in 1995 reported the National Institutes of Neurological Disorders and Stroke(NINDS) tPA stroke trial. (1) The trial demonstrated that intravenous thrombolysis with tissue plasminogen activator (tPA) improved recovery in stroke patients treated within three hours of stroke onset. This was the first demonstration that medication given intravenously could dissolve a clot causing stroke, resulting in improvement of the stroke. A direct attack on the problem of patients having a stroke was finally available. The day of the "Clot-Buster" had arrived.

tPA generated fresh interest in stroke care in the medical and neurology community. At last, there was something to do when a stroke occurred. This prompted the development of systems to provide rapid therapy for ischemic stroke therapy. Standards for certification of a Primary Stroke Center were published in December 2003. Primary certification was centered on intra-venous treatment and did not require extensive capability in neuro-intervention and neurosurgery. Dr. David Wang of the INI, very early on, developed the largest rural stroke network system, eventually involving 26 hospitals, thus forming the first certified Primary Stroke Center in Illinois. His objective: patients in rural areas would consistently receive prompt state-of-the-art stroke treatment.

With treatment available, early recognition of stroke by patients, families, and ambulance and emergency room staff was critical. People working in Newcastle UK developed in 1998, a FAST acronym (Face, Arms, Speech, Telephone) to remind people of stroke assessment and to get them to call 911 rather than procrastinate or take steps that will not immediately lead to stroke care. The OSF HealthCare stoke service held many public meet-ings and worked with ambulance services and emergency rooms throughout Illinois delivering the FAST message. FAST posters were painted on the sides of ambulances, and awareness of stroke changed dramatically in several years.

More demanding requirements were addressed nine years later with Comprehensive Stroke Center Certification by the Joint Commission in September 2012. (2, 11, 12) This document provided a benchmark for the elements of a comprehensive cerebrovascular center and is an excellent reference document. This new level of care requires 24/7/365 consistent high-quality stroke imaging, evaluation, and care by vascular neurologists, availability of vascular neurosurgery specialists, and endovas-cular neuro-interventionalists. These services are supported by a neurological critical care unit and specialized nurses in the critical care unit and acute neurology floor.

Emergency Medical Systems (EMS) have treatment guide-lines in place and are staffed by emergency physicians familiar with modern stroke care. Well trained ambulance staff are a critical initial entrance to the treatment process. There are outlined requirements to assure timely entrance to an appropriately staffed endovascular laboratory, or a neurovascular surgery operating room. The importance of well-developed stroke rehabilitation is addressed. APN's support care and provide follow up in a comprehensive center.

Because comprehensive centers require a remarkable concentration of skilled specialists, they have a responsibility to society to contribute to the understanding of stroke and improved care. A clinical research program with participation in multi-center trials is essential.

September 21, 2012, the Illinois Neurological Institute was the second in the United States to achieve certification as a Comprehensive Stroke Center. The INI Stroke and cerebrovascular group, led by Dr. David Wang, already had assembled the necessary infrastructure, the ICU, vascular neurosurgery, and endovascular services in the preceding decade. Our Comprehensive Stroke Center offers the full spectrum of care, at all times. Today, comprehensive centers are achieving significant improvements in disability prevention, return to home, and to full activity in patients experiencing a stroke.

The comprehensive center added timely neuro-interventional intra-arterial clot removal to the standards, the care that saved Ralph Black from lifelong disability. The scientific validation of this intervention was delivered in four studies reported in early 2015, three years after the establishment of comprehensive stroke centers. A randomized trial of intra-arterial treatment for acute ischemic stroke published in the *New England Journal of Medicine* reported experience with early intra-arterial thrombolysis in proximal intracranial occlusion in the anterior circulation (MR CLEAN Trial). This was the first study directly extracting the clot from the occluded carotid or middle cerebral artery and establishing the value of intra-arterial thrombolysis over intravenous thrombolysis. Compared to intravenous thrombolysis, it provided a 13.5 percent improvement improvement in functional independence.

Two studies were published immediately in the *New England Journal of Medicine*, the EXTEND-IA Trial from Australia and the ESCAPE trial, a larger multinational trial, both closing early because of proof of efficacy. Both studies excluded patients with large infarcts (strokes) by CT angiography and CT perfusion studies. Excluding patients that clearly would not be benefited by treatment created a much improved trial design. In a short time, three large studies demonstrated the superiority of endovascular therapy in carotid and M 1 occlusion. (3, 4, 5) This evidence challenged healthcare systems to develop a rapid triage system with a comprehensive stroke center offering experienced endovascular thrombosis management with time limits of 3-4.5 hours.

In early 2018, further change occurred with a report in the *New England Journal of Medicine* indicating that intra-arterial thrombectomy could be done as late as 24 hours in patients where a specialized perfusion CT scan revealed that a significant amount of viable brain remained well beyond the previous time limit. (13, 14). These two studies, DAWN and INFUSE 3 resulted in a further change in stroke guidelines challenging medical systems to identify and arrange care for another subset of stroke patients. Computer software applying artificial intelligence is used to rapidly identify patients with remaining salvageable brain tissue making them candidates for immediate transfer to an endovascular laboratory for thrombectomy. RAPID is used in the INI Comprehensive Stroke Center to rapidly identify these patients. Several other companies have products in development (Viz.ai and Neural Analytics Inc.) (15)

Demonstrated efficacy of intra-arterial treatment demands a changed care process in a multi-hospital stroke system. Scientific evidence generates a major administrative challenge to provide the care in systems. Because of endovascular expertise manpower constraints and cost structure, a health system will probably have one or two Comprehensive Stroke Centers leading a system program. Most associated small and medium-size hospitals fulfill requirements for Primary Stroke Center. A significant shortage of general neurologists requires the development of treatment protocols in the ER and acute medical floors working with emergency room physicians and hospitalists. TeleNeurology can provide vascular neurology expertise. This level of care involves the development of transfer mechanisms for patients needing immediate treatment by a neuro-interventionalist or neurosurgeon. Patients must be brought to the right place, at the right time, consistently.

Primary stroke centers have made progress in prompt thrombolysis in patients presenting within the IV thrombolysis window (the period when the "clot-buster" tPA can be safely given intravenously) which has recently been extended from 3.0 to 4.5 hours. Recently, an ambulance (Mobile Stroke Unit MSU) equipped with a CT scanner and staffed with a neurologist was put in place at Charite Hospital Berlin to increase the opportunity for tPA to be administered within the "Golden Hour". A similar program has been initiated at Memorial Hermann hospital in Houston, USA. (6, 8) The Memorial Hermann program provides the Mobile Stroke Unit (MSU) alternating weekly with current standard care to investigate the potential benefit of MSU in management. The study also is investigating the value of a TeleNeurology vascular neurologist in this process. Houston has 3 Comprehensive Stroke Centers, and stroke management is a regional priority. At the CSC's 14% of patients and 90% of tPA eligible patients were treated with tPA within 3 hours. As many more mobile stroke units develop, experience will determine if this is an appropriate direction in stroke care.

Improving time from onset of symptoms to patient's

presentation for care remains a challenge. Mobile stroke units may be one solution, but improving patient and family awareness of stroke symptoms, the urgency of treatment, and the importance of arriving at the optimum site for treatment, is a less technically challenging and less expensive solution meriting further study. We have to target those at risk and increase the awareness of stroke treatment of patients at risk and their families. Electronic medical record software can identify the population at risk for targeted office education. Those at risk should not leave their doctor's office without stroke education and a refrigerator magnet.

Substantial progress has been made in the treatment of hemorrhagic cerebral vascular disease; intracerebral hematoma, aneurysm, and arteriovenous malformation. Optimally, patients with subarachnoid hemorrhage caused by an aneurysm need to be evaluated, in the early hours after hemorrhage, by both a neuro-interventionalist and a vascular neurosurgeon, for appropriate treatment offering lasting protection from rehemorrhage with low morbidity. This involves the availability of high levels of expertise in microsurgery and endovascular intervention at all times.

Neuro-interventionalist coiling and neurosurgical clipping of aneurysms, and management of arteriovenous malformations require significant continuing experience for optimum care with low morbidity. Multiple recent publications have demonstrated a relationship between volume and outcome. Most healthcare systems require a single destination center with these capabilities. A modern endovascular room costs approximately $5.0 million with an extensive inventory of coils, stents, catheters, and embolic agents costing more than $1.0 million. Comprehensive Stroke Center designation requires 24/7 technical staffing. Cost and maintenance of physician and staff competence make replication of units unfeasible. Small health care systems require contracting and transportation arrangements with a comprehensive center to achieve high-quality care at an acceptable cost.

Strong evidence of benefit from the evacuation of intracerebral hematoma (blood clot in brain substance) does not exist. New work with less invasive methods of clot removal utilizing advanced imaging to visualize deep white matter fiber pathways suggests new approaches. The goal; remove the clot without producing new brain damage in the process. These technological improvements may make intracerebral hematoma removal a superior management, just as technological improvement changed intra-arterial clot removal.

Patients are now being enrolled in a phase III randomized case-controlled, open-label 500 subject clinical trial of minimally invasive surgery plus tPA in the treatment of intracerebral hemorrhage (MISTIE III). Daniel Hanley M.D. of Johns Hopkins University is the NIH sponsored Study Chair. The study has an anticipated completion date of September 2019, with final enrollment in September 2018. (7) Studies utilizing a minimally invasive subcortical parafascicular access for clot evacuation (Mi SPACE) employ new fascicular (white matter fiber pathways) imaging techniques to minimize the neurological invasiveness of the process. A path to the clot is designed to avoid injury to deep brain pathways by passing through white matter with less critical function. If positive, these studies will support the transfer of intracerebral hemorrhage patients to centers with cerebrovascular neurosurgery expertise requiring further alteration of current care patterns.

Many stroke patients benefit from specialized care in a center, and this challenges patient transfer, process design, and culture change in health systems. The functional and cognitive benefits are so high that achievement is imperative. Patients and families must be more aware of what they must do, and hospital systems must be forthright about their ability to provide necessary state-of-the-art care. Optimum care in stroke is changing by the year, steadily providing new logistical challenges. Each stroke patient should receive the same opportunity to avoid disability experienced by Ralph Black. This represents a very significant logistical challenge in rural America.

Balance and Vertigo

When a vigorous elderly person experiences a fall, it is often the first step to disability, a nursing home, and loss of independent existence. With an active aging population, problems of dizziness, balance, and vertigo have become a challenge in population health care. Over 2.4 million Americans over age 65 were treated in emergency departments after falls in 2012, and, each year, about 25,000 die after falls. Falls are multifactorial, and impaired balance in the elderly is a major factor. Assessment of balance and fall risk should be an integral part of an office visit in the elderly, and risk counseling and referral for a balance program is often advisable. Balance evaluation and training programs are provided in our physical therapy departments, allowing this service to be available near patient's homes. A balance program for the elderly can delay admission to a nursing home or assisted living facility.

A recent study estimates that 35 percent of adults aged 40 years or older, in the United States, have experienced some form of balance or vestibular dysfunction. The National Institute on Deafness and Other Communication Disorders (NIDCD) reports that 4 percent of American adults report chronic balance problems, with an additional 2.4 million reporting chronic dizziness. Vertigo and dizziness lead to over 4 million emergency department visits and admissions annually at a cost of $9 billion. Millions of dollars are spent on imaging to detect the small percentage of patients with life-threatening posterior fossa strokes and brain tumor presenting as dizziness.

Rapidly differentiating relatively minor, easily treated balance problems from serious brain disease is a major public health problem. Emergency Department physicians rank vertigo a top priority for development of improved diagnostic techniques. Patients with vestibular neuritis and benign paroxysmal vertigo (not life-threatening) often undergo unnecessary imaging studies in emergency rooms and then, are admitted to the hospital. At the same time, some patients with dangerous brain stem or cerebellar strokes are sent home. (1, 2, 3, 5)

A spectrum of chronic and acute balance conditions require evaluation and care in a large health care system:

1. Benign paroxysmal positional vertigo
2. Bilateral loss of labyrinthine function
3. Labyrinthitis
4. Meniere's disease
5. Vestibular migraine

In addition to this well-defined group of vestibular illnesses, many patients develop symptoms involving gait disturbance (walking imbalance) and various rather subjective symptoms of unsteadiness requiring evaluation. These patients often have inappropriate and expensive studies and less than adequate management. Development of a system of care beginning with the initial primary care visit presents a challenge for healthcare systems.

Benign paroxysmal positional vertigo (BPPV) is a common, suddenly developing problem experienced by the middle-aged and elderly population. BPPV is a mechanical inner ear problem that occurs when the otoliths (calcium carbonate crystals) are displaced into one of the semicircular canals of the inner ear, changing fluid movement. This results in false signals sent to the brain. Patients with BPPV receive relief with repositioning techniques (neck movement positioning) that return the otoliths to the utricle. Prompt recognition leads to appropriate treatment without extensive and expensive testing.

Kerber reported on 3522 ER visits for dizziness in Nueces County Texas, from 2008 to 2011. (4) He found that a Dix-Hallpike test (a test for BPPV) had been done in only 137 visits (3.9 percent) and that an otolith repositioning maneuver (CRM, Epley maneuver movement of the head and neck-a repositioning treatment for BVVP) had been done in 8 visits (0.2 percent). Diagnosis of BPPV was made in 156 visits (4.4 percent), indicating that doctors, nurses, and the patients were unaware of the condition, its diagnosis, and relatively easy treatment. An unnecessary head CT was done in 1,162 visits (33 percent). If BPPV is not appropriately identified, CT scanning and prolonged ER visits result, leading to patients experiencing the discomfort and expense of unnecessary testing, without relief of their problem. Cost of care created without value for the patient.

Repositioning care is provided by audiologists, neurologists, or a specialty nurse. Emergency room physicians are gradually acquiring this skill. A healthcare system in a metropolitan area can offer a nurse staffed clinic to teach the Epley maneuver, avoiding the need to teach this expertise in multiple physician offices, where it is used infrequently. CT and MRI scanning are unnecessary in BPPV. Exclusion of serious stroke from cerebellar hemorrhage, and brain stem infarction from posterior inferior cerebellar or vertebral artery disease is necessary and usually can be differentiated by clinical evaluation. A well- designed care path for acute vertigo syndromes will ultimately support this process in primary care offices, Prompt Care(urgent care), and emergency care facilities.

To support the health care system, a point of intake into specialized care for the remaining complex problems is provided by the INI Balance Center, providing the services of a specialty vestibular neurologist, audiologists, otologist, balance rehabilitation staff, and neurosurgeons. The center provides evaluation for complex problems, and advice to physicians in the management of illnesses, not requiring travel to the referral center. The center offers a number of specialized studies when needed: audiometric testing, caloric testing, electro-oculography, electronystagmography, posturography, vestibular-evoked myogenic potentials and vestibular function testing with a rotary chair with computer analysis of nystagmus and extra-ocular movements.

Epilepsy

Early in my career, poorly controlled seizures were a common problem in the emergency room. Treatment was limited to intravenous barbiturates and Dilantin. Surgery was rarely offered to patients with intractable temporal lobe seizures, at that time. Reading about Dr. Penfield's pioneering epilepsy research in Montreal drew me to neurosurgery. I was part of the pioneering program in temporal lobe epilepsy surgery with Dr. Percival Bailey and Dr. Fred Gibbs in Chicago. Years of dedicated work by epilepsy investigators have not led to universal effective epilepsy care.

One in ten people will have a seizure during their life, and a significant number have further seizures and receive a diagnosis of epilepsy. There are 500 new epilepsy cases diagnosed daily in the United States, 200,000 per year; 30% are children, and 2.3 million adults have epilepsy. Delayed diagnosis and inadequate treatment continue to lead to further seizures, disability, job loss, falls, injury, and occasionally death. Of 2.7 million Americans with epilepsy, approximately 25-30% have inadequate seizure control and suffer from intractable epilepsy.

In Ontario, Canada between 2001 and 2010, 10,661 patients were identified with medically intractable epilepsy. (1) Only 124 patients (1.2 %) underwent epilepsy surgery within 2 years of being defined as medically intractable. Death occurred in 12

% of those with medically intractable epilepsy. One-quarter of adults with active epilepsy reported not taking any medicine to control their seizure disorder. One third of adults reported physical disability/inability to work compared to a small proportion of the general population. Half of the patients reporting active epilepsy were receiving Social Security disability payment. Most patients were able to obtain medical care, yet continued to have active epilepsy and a significant number were not taking medication. This population experience clearly defines a problem, not effectively addressed by our health system.

Advances in diagnosis, medical management, and epilepsy surgery are inadequately utilized by treating physicians, and the public, resulting in patients achieving less than optimum seizure control. This may be one of the more glaring deficiencies in "population medicine". The concept of "one seizure is too many" should be embedded in national medical practice. Healthcare systems need to identify patients and make them aware of the potential benefit of decreased disability and unemployment achieved with medical management. The complaisance of physicians and health administrators regarding our care of patients experiencing seizures troubles me. It certainly has not received the attention afforded to stroke. Seizure medications are not the subject of repetitive TV advertisements.

Most patients with epilepsy can be managed by their primary care physician or general neurologist, considered the first and second levels of epilepsy care. Patients having persistent seizures or subsequent side effects should be considered to have failed standard treatment and should be referred without delay to a third or fourth level specialty epilepsy center. The National Association of Epilepsy Centers developed criteria for Level Three and Four centers. (2)

These centers have:

1. An interdisciplinary care team approach

2. Electrodiagnostic facilities
3. Safety protocols and quality measures
4. Patient education

The interdisciplinary care team is led by a neurologist or neurosurgeon with special expertise and interest in epilepsy. A video-EEG monitoring unit is needed for evaluation, as well as specialized brain imaging and cognitive testing. Qualified EEG technicians and specialized nursing staff are critical. The American Academy of Neurology (AAN) has developed a number of quality measures for seizure care.

A Level 3 Epilepsy Center provides the basic range of medical, neuropsychological, and psychosocial services needed to treat patients with refractory epilepsy. These centers also offer noninvasive evaluation for epilepsy surgery, straightforward epilepsy resective surgery (often a specific lesion resection or an anterior temporal lobectomy in mesial temporal sclerosis), and implantation of vagus nerve stimulators. Intracranial grid monitoring evaluations or more complex resective epilepsy surgery are not performed.

Grid monitoring requires a craniotomy with placement of a sheet of recording electrodes (grid) directly on the brain, to precisely localize the site of seizure origin. The wound is closed with wires that are connected to the grid exiting the scalp in a single cable. After grid placement, the patient is observed and recorded in a monitoring unit for several days. Precise localization of the origin of the seizure is obtained. Stimulation testing permits analysis of brain function in the area underlying the grid. The epileptologist and neurosurgeon must have two years of experience, and perform a minimum of 50 video EEG monitoring cases per year.

The INI has a Level 4 Epilepsy Center providing complex intensive neurodiagnostic monitoring and extensive medical, neuropsychological and psychosocial treatment. Level 4 centers offer a complete evaluation for epilepsy surgery, including intracranial electrode recording, a broad range of surgical procedures for epilepsy, and clinical trials. Functional cortical mapping by stimulation of subdural electrodes, either extra-operatively (while in the monitoring unit) or intraoperatively is provided. These facilities allow precise identification of function in areas considered for removal and relates these critical areas to the site of seizure origin. Often, information provided by intracranial electrodes leads to resection of epileptogenic tissue in the absence of obvious structural lesions such as brain tumors and arteriovenous malformations. The center offers specialized neuroimaging either on-site or by established arrangement including interictal (between seizures) PET and/or ictal (during seizures) SPECT scans. Although there is no absolute number of surgeries, at least 100 cases should be evaluated annually to assure continued competence of the staff.

A health care system needs to provide excellent care for seizure patients and support caretakers. Inadequate care leads to repeated visits to emergency rooms, repeated and inappropriate imaging, and disability and loss of employment for the patients and families involved. Although much of the care can be provided by primary care and general neurology, recognition of inadequate control and prompt referral for expert care is essential. A large system can develop a Level 3 or Level 4 center if the system serves a population large enough to generate the volume necessary to maintain staff expertise. Developing the business case is difficult; the immense personal and financial benefit of the patient's return to a productive role in society is not included in the formula.

If center development is not feasible, a relationship to a Level 4 epilepsy center should be established. Level 3 or 4 centers develop protocols or care paths with the physician medical group for investigation and care of seizure disorders, to validate medical management, imaging and diagnostic evaluation. Educational programs for primary care physicians and APN's assure all patients have an opportunity for optimum seizure management. (3, 4) Inappropriate use of CT scanning instead of well-designed MRI studies for seizure investigation, acceptance of imperfect seizure control, and extensive use of emergency rooms continue to be opportunities for improvement in most healthcare systems. It is estimated that only one person in ten that would benefit from epilepsy surgery has the procedure performed in the United States. The center assumes responsibility for population health in epilepsy.

There remains a reluctance in general medicine and general neurology to promptly identify inadequate control and refer for surgical evaluation. OSF HealthCare continues development of protocols to identify patients who would benefit from further evaluation and care in a specialty center. I walked into Penfield's Montreal Neurological Institute 60 years ago; the progress in the care of those suffering from epilepsy is not a basis for complacency.

Although epilepsy population care eludes us, exciting less invasive surgical techniques are in development. Stereo-EEG (SEEG), placing multiple depth electrodes robotically, enhances diagnosis in complex problems. Placement of laser energy in a seizure focus with intraoperative MRI guidance is now being done, to achieve obliteration of an identified seizure focus without craniotomy. Stimulators are being placed in the brain to actively monitor the brain's electrical activity, and stimulate the brain when specific seizure patterns appear, stopping further seizure development. Thus, the patient is not disturbed by a clinical seizure. This technique is being utilized in patients with medically uncontrolled seizures not amenable to surgical resection. (5) The challenge to American medicine is the application of these new developments across the broad population.

20 Years of Intense Right Facial Pain Solution Needed

Richard Smith, a 55-year-old construction worker, had severe pain in the right cheek and eye for an hour or more each day, for 15 days, without relief. His history was long and complicated. The first episode occurred twenty years before, lasting six weeks, and he had similar episodes, one or two times a year, after that. Each episode began with right-sided nasal stuffiness, right eye tearing, followed by intense pain behind the right eye. He saw multiple neurologists and took various medications, always with only partial relief. Richard achieved some improvement with medications for migraine headache and cluster headache. Cluster headache is a relatively rare headache that occurs in clusters lasting 4-8 weeks. They are always one-sided, usually causing severe pain in back of the eye, and are more common in men. Richard's MRI was normal, and my impression was that he was suffering from cluster headache.

Richard, in the past, responded to Sumatriptan medication and had taken Verapamil for prevention, but recently, these medications failed to help. When first seen, he was three weeks into a cluster. After 20 years, Richard had lost patience with organized medicine and was exploring all alternatives on the internet. He was aware that a few patients had been successfully treated with Gamma Knife radiation of the nerves involved. The reported work described delivering a high dose of radiation to the spheno-palatine ganglion in the skull base and, to the fifth nerve, before it enters the brain. Both nerves are believed to be involved in the production of a cluster headache.

After several visits with Richard, a Gamma Knife treatment was arranged, with Richard understanding that treatment was investigational. The morning of the procedure, I attached a Leksell stereotactic frame to his head with four small pins with local anesthesia. He then had an MRI and a CT scan relating the markers on the frame to the targets in his skull and brain. I developed a plan to deliver a dose of 90 Gy radiation to the sphenopalatine ganglion, in the lower two-thirds of his pterygopalatine fossa, just in back and above the nose, in the base of the skull. An 80 Gy dose of radiation was delivered to the fifth cranial nerve (trigeminal nerve) before it enters the brain stem.

The Gamma Knife is very precise, so we could assure that the eyes, the optic nerves, and the brain would not receive significant radiation. All of this took most of the morning, starting at 5:30 a.m., so he returned home that afternoon and returned to work the next day. The effect of this radiation usually occurs over weeks or months, so we continued to treat this cluster with his medicines, and the headaches ceased in two weeks.

Richard had a mild episode a year later lasting two weeks and has not had subsequent clusters. Additional work in this area has been published, but conclusive evidence of efficacy of radiation in cluster headache is not established. In the interim, new work has been reported using an embedded stimulator, at the sphenopalatine ganglion, to stop headaches. Management of a disabling headache continues to require dedicated persistence and clinical expertise, with a few patients needing the support of a specialty center.

Headache

Headache is an important population health problem, creating great disability and patient suffering. The World Health Organization ranks migraine as the 19th cause of disability, with 6-8 % of men and 15-18 % of women experiencing migraine. In the United States, 3000 migraine attacks occur per million people, per day. In the United Kingdom, 25 million working or school days are lost, per year, to headache. Headache spending in the United States reached $2.8 billion and neuroimaging for headache in the United States between 2007 and 2010 approached $1.2 billion. Tension-type headache is a recurring problem in numerous patients, with a peak in the '30s, followed in frequency by various other types of chronic daily headache. Cluster headache as experienced by Richard, although infrequent, is a source of great suffering and episodic disability.

The INI Headache Center provides care for migraine, tension-type headache, chronic headache syndromes, and cluster headache. Dr. Hrachya Nersesyan, the neurologist leading the program serves a diagnostic and therapeutic role for complex headache management. Hrachya trained in neurosurgery at the Burdenko Neurosurgical Institute in Moscow, then came to the United States, where he did a fellowship in functional neurosurgery, then a neurology residency at the INI. He has an intense commitment to improving the care of headache. Physicians with this interest and commitment are unfortunately extremely scarce. His clinic team includes an advanced practice nurse, a neuropsychologist and a social worker. Dr. Nersesyan intends to develop a low-light, quiet room for short-term infusion therapy, with an infusion clinic available 12 hours a day, avoiding emergency and prompt care use for a substantial portion of the patients. Development awaits administrative space and budget commitment. This approach will provide improved care with decreased cost.

Dr. Nersesyan is developing, in collaboration with primary care medicine, protocols and educational programs to improve the ability of primary care physicians to provide management of the large headache population. Primary care providers can manage a significant portion of the patients after initial diagnosis and recommendations, allowing the headache specialty team to see both new patients and established complex patients in a timely fashion.

The population health challenge; cost-effective evaluation, diagnosis avoiding unnecessary imaging, decreasing headache associated disability, and decreasing repeated trips to emergency rooms and prompt care facilities. E.R. visits often result in inappropriate repetitive imaging with CT and MRI. A health care system must address these problems. Appropriate investigation of a headache is a major factor in patient convenience and cost. Loder et al. in "Choosing Wisely in Headache Medicine: The American Headache Society's List of Five Things Physicians and Patients Should Question" discourages neuroimaging in patients with stable headaches that meet criteria for a migraine. "Choosing Wisely" guidelines by the American College of Radiology and Consumer Reports also suggested: "Don't do imaging for uncomplicated headaches."(1) Most published guidelines suggest that neuroimaging should be ordered only if a stable headache patient displays localizing neurological signs or symptoms.

Dr. A. H. Hawasli, at Washington University, approached the problem from the perspective of physicians seeing patients with brain tumor. (2) His study illustrates the dilemma in dealing with conditions with significant morbidity such as brain tumor that is relatively rare in large populations. A retrospective study of patients revealed to have a brain tumor on open biopsy, showed 11.6% had only isolated headache. Concern that these tumors will be missed is the cause of a great deal of brain imaging in headache patients. Headache patients fear they harbor a brain tumor and demand imaging, often an MRI.

A large healthcare system requires an inpatient service for intractable headache, status migrainosus, medication overuse and rebound, and complicated secondary headache. We have not met this challenge in the INI. This requires an identified section of the acute neurology floor staffed with nurses possessing specialized headache knowledge. The unit would be a resource for the entire health system. Creation of an inpatient unit requires planning and relationships with major payers. Payers must be assured that decreased cost and less disability will result. The neuropsychology support for this unit would also serve the outpatient clinic. Scale supporting recruitment and retention of scarce neuropsychologists is achieved. An inpatient headache unit will support a busy destination outpatient headache center.

Honeymoon, Happiness, and then Dementia

Elizabeth Kunkle had a wonderful career as an eighth-grade teacher and retired rather late at 72. She was career oriented and never married. In retirement, she met a widower on an organized community outing, and over time, they grew fond of one another and married, taking a long honeymoon cruise. Within months of their return, Elizabeth became forgetful, leaving items on the stove to burn, and other dangerous activities. Her husband Ed was puzzled and decimated after a diagnosis of Alzheimer's was made. Because he was unable to assure her safety, she was admitted to an assisted living facility. Ed visited daily, providing support but Elizabeth became bedridden over several months and continued to regress.

One evening, Elizabeth fell while getting from her bed to the bathroom without waiting for assistance, striking her head. She was sent to an emergency room outside of Peoria, where she was found to be drowsy, confused, with no apparent arm or leg paralysis. A CT scan was done, and she was transferred to Saint Francis Medical Center. I was asked to see her that night. Elizabeth was drowsy, but answered simple questions and followed simple commands. Her memory and ability to follow instructions were impaired. The CT scan did not reveal any evidence of injury but did show a massive frontal lobe tumor. An olfactory groove meningioma, a benign tumor, was growing out of the base of the skull, above the nose. I advised surgery, telling the patient and her husband that the degree of recovery was unpredictable.

Several days later, I made an incision in back of her hairline, opened the skull of the forehead on both sides, and, over 4 -5 hours, removed a massive tumor from the skull base. The tumor extended to the optic nerves and chiasm but did not involve them. With the microscope, I was able to easily remove the tumor next to the optic nerves and carotid arteries. After surgery, she awakened slowly, and gradually became stronger and more alert, and was able to return to the nursing home in seven days. Elizabeth could maintain a conversation at the first office visit, but her thoughts lacked organization. She was not ready to return to their home, but she and Ed were hopeful. Because they lived at some distance, I arranged for further follow up with their physician, planning to see her in one year.

Four months later, I received a postcard from her husband Ed. They were on a cruise, and he felt she was very much like when they were married. Dementia had been conquered.

As the population ages, changes in cognition and dementia are more common, and not all patients have such a pleasing outcome. Nevertheless, there are treatable forms of dementia, and exciting preventive measures and treatments, on the horizon. Much of the care for patients with cognitive decline can be provided in the community, but specialized evaluation is sometimes needed to identify treatable problems or to give patients and families an accurate prognosis.

Cognitive Disorders and Brain Health

Disorders of cognition leading to dementia are an increasing health problem with the aging of our population. Measured in disability years, it is a greater cause of disability than stroke, neuromuscular disease, cardiovascular disease, and cancer. Disordered cognition disables the patient, and requires support either from family or outside resources, generating further economic and social cost. In 2015, care of Alzheimer's and other dementias cost the US economy $226 billion. A health system is obliged to provide a memory and brain health program to ameliorate the social and economic cost of cognitive disease.

With increased public awareness, fear of Alzheimer's disease is a growing problem. Elderly people live in fear of "becoming a vegetable" and ending their lives in a nursing home. With increasing lifespan, the incidence of dementia is progressively higher with age, generating stress and escalating cost. Recent publications, hopefully, suggest a possible decrease in incidence. Review of data from the Framingham Heart Study is encouraging. (1, 2) The Framingham Heart Study is a community based, longitudinal cohort study that was initiated in 1948, involving 5209 residents of Framingham, Massachusetts. In 1971, 5214 offspring of the participants in the original cohort were enrolled.

The dementia study involved 5205 people 60 years or older, under surveillance for dementia since 1975. The study revealed that the 5 year age and sex-adjusted cumulative hazard rates for dementia were 3.6 per 100 persons during the first epoch (late 1970s and early 1980s), 2.8 per 100 persons during the second epoch (late 1980s and early 1990s), 2.2 per 100 persons during the third epoch (late 1990s and early 2000s), and 2.0 per 100 persons during the fourth epoch (late 2000s and early 2010s). They further observed that there was a trend toward an increasing mean age at diagnosis, from 80 years, during the first epoch, to 85 years during the fourth epoch. Risk reduction occurred only in those with at least a high school diploma. Although vascular risk factors decreased during that time, the study authors felt that they failed to entirely explain the decrease in risk of dementia. This encouraging change may moderate the societal stress associated with increasing life span. Langa et al. in a study utilizing data from the Health and Retirement Study (HRS) compared the prevalence of dementia in the United States in 2000 and 2012. They found the incidence in people over 65 years falling from 11.6% to 8.8% in the 12-year interval, also finding the relationship between educational attainment and decrease in dementia. (3)

Treatment is not anticipated to restore lost function. If medication benefitting dementia becomes available, diagnosis, before significant symptoms occur, will be necessary. The race for an identifying biomarker permitting early diagnosis has started. We may face a period when we can definitively diagnose the disease, and identify a treatment that is efficacious, but treatment will have started too late to provide a meaningful benefit for those identified. If treatment must be started before the onset of symptoms, a generation of patients may be diagnosed, without future benefit from treatment. A biomarker, indicating the presence of the illness before clinical symptoms, will have great value only when effective treatment may be offered.

The INI Memory and Brain Health Center provides comprehensive evaluation and consultation. Development of a system-wide supportive care structure is an ultimate goal. (4) Dr. Biernot, INI cognitive neurologist, led a small team including an advanced practice nurse, a neuropsychologist, and a social worker. Evaluation sometimes leads to specific treatment after identification of treatable dementia. More often the cognitive decline will not have specific medical treatment, and supportive care prolongs independent living and decreases family stress. Patients present in a number of categories: mild cognitive impairment, rapidly progressing dementia, dementia in the relatively young, Alzheimer's, and non-Alzheimer's dementias. The prevalence rate of dementia is 1.4 percent ages 65-69, 2.8 percent ages 70-74, 5.6 percent ages 75-79, 10.5 percent ages 80-84, 20.8 percent at 85-89, and 38.6 percent at 90-94 years.

Patients with early onset, rapidly progressive dementia or atypical symptoms should be seen by cognitive neurologists in a memory and brain health center for prompt initial consultation and evaluation. There are a host of identifiable treatable and non-treatable causes of dementia: Creutzfeldt-Jakob disease (a prion disease), infectious diseases, human immunodeficiency virus infection, progressive multifocal leukoencephalopathy, cryptococcal infection, and other viral and fungus infections, auto-immune disorders, paraneoplastic disorders, and metabolic disorders (hepatic encephalopathy, vitamin deficiencies including Vitamin B 12 and thiamine, and hypothyroidism).

Normal pressure hydrocephalous (NPH), a defect in cerebrospinal fluid absorption, must be considered if urinary incontinence and gait ataxia are present. Hydrocephalous shunt insertion sometimes leads to striking clinical improvement. Since shunt insertion has a number of associated complications, patient selection is critical and challenging.

More slowly progressing dementia in patients over 65 is most frequently Alzheimer's disease. Vascular dementia, frontotemporal dementia, and Lewy Body Dementia comprise those 35% of patients that do not have Alzheimer's disease.

All patients have a baseline mental state evaluation such as the Kokmen Short Test of Mental Status or the Folstein Mini-Mental State Examination. Many need formal neuropsychological testing to establish a baseline, determine the cognitive domains impaired, assess for depression, and subsequently determine progression. This takes several hours and requires a skilled neuropsychologist. MRI is useful in the evaluation of normal pressure hydrocephalous, vascular dementia, and brain tumor.

PET scanning for beta-amyloid is now readily available, but quite expensive, and usually not covered by insurance plans. It is not diagnostic, but the absence of amyloid on scan excludes Alzheimer's disease as a diagnosis. The Centers for Medicare and Medicaid Services (CMS) in 2015 began a multicenter national study "Imaging Dementia — Evidence for Amyloid Scanning"

(IDEAS) to determine the effect of amyloid PET imaging on management. Currently, amyloid testing is considered in the face of a cognitive complaint with objectively confirmed impairment, and the diagnosis remains uncertain upon comprehensive evaluation by a dementia expert. Pet scan is often utilized in evaluating those under 65 years old with progressive dementia. It should not be utilized in patients with cognitive complaints without clinical confirmation of impairment.

Genetic testing currently has limited application in cognitive disorders. Testing is available for Autosomal Dominant Alzheimer's Disease, which accounts for less than 5% of the patients with Alzheimer's disease, usually with a clear family history and early onset. The presence of polymorphism, of the apolipoprotein E (ApoE) gene, specifically the ApoE4 allele, greatly increases the risk of developing dementia. Almost 25% of the population who have one or two copies of this allele do not develop dementia. This makes testing of limited value and potentially damaging to the patient's sense of well-being.

The INI Memory and Brain Health Center supports the care of patients in the healthcare system, with a particular responsibility for evaluating those with early onset or rapid progression. The center is developing protocols for physicians to evaluate and initiate care for the large portion of patients with late-onset disease and less challenging management. This allows prompt evaluation and initiation of care for most patients. The center staff continues to play a significant role in the management of patients with Lewy Body dementia and frontotemporal dementias, because these patients need continued complex medical management. The center, through coordination of the work of social workers, neuropsychologists, and advanced practice nurses, enhances the life and function of patients with dementia and their families. The national shortage of neurologists specializing in cognitive disorders results in inordinate delay in initial evaluation, and lack of adequate continued support for those patients with complex dementia syndromes requiring consultant support. The INI, like other centers, needs twice as many cognitive neurologists and neuropsychologists as it is possible to recruit.

Recently, Dr. Biernot moved to Boston accompanying her husband. Coping with the remarkable shortage of cognitive neurologists, the INI began a teleneurology program utilizing an experienced cognitive APN in Peoria, with Dr. Biernot performing consultation and monitoring management at a distance. This system could provide excellent care and allow us to develop a novel delivery system, but for our lack of cognitive neurologists and neuropsychologists. It is a chilling reminder of the national shortage in this subspecialty that remains to be addressed by academic leadership.

The National Institute on Aging funds twenty-nine Alzheimer's disease centers in the United States. Although each center has an area of research emphasis, a common goal is to enhance research by creating a network that shares new ideas, expertise, and research results. The centers draw upon the expertise of scientists in multiple disciplines. The aging demographics of the United States make this an important focus in a time of limited resources, and a substantial responsibility for the INI. Clinicians in the INI Memory and Brain Health Center must work with investigators in the University of Illinois College Of Medicine to improve the understanding of degenerative brain disease and to better identify diagnostic markers and measures of disease activity.

In a destination cognition outpatient center, co-location with the movement disorders center and the multiple sclerosis center allows joint utilization of physical therapy, occupational therapy, social work, neuropsychology and gait laboratory.

Parkinson's Disease and Movement Disorders

Movement disorders include a group of neurological illnesses that impair the regulation of voluntary motor movement without directly impairing strength, and usually result from dysfunction in gray matter structures deep in the brain termed the basal ganglia. This diverse illness group is cared for by subspecialty movement disorder neurologists. Although Parkinson's disease is the dominant disorder, a movement disorder neurologist also cares for patients with essential tremor, athetosis, dystonia, and multiple system disease.

Parkinson's disease incidence increases with aging, with an incidence of 93 per 100,000 in the 70- to 79-year-old group. One million Americans live with Parkinson's disease and related syndromes, with an estimated cost including treatment, social security payments, and lost income from work disability of nearly $25 billion per year. Medication costs average $2,500 per year and Deep Brain Stimulation (DBS) surgery can cost up to $100,000 per patient. Michael Kinsley provides a very personal insight of Parkinson's disease in *Old Age: A Beginner's Guide.* (1)

With the aging of our population, assisting these patients is a meaningful challenge to families and health care systems. Movement disorders have a broad spectrum of symptoms, generate significant disability, and have benefitted from new medical and deep brain stimulation treatments, making a comprehensive treatment program essential.

In 1958, before the availability of medical management with L-3, 4-dihydroxyphenylalanine (levodopa, L-Dopa), I performed stereotactic operations for Parkinson's tremor in Chicago one day a week. Lesions in the globus pallidus or the ventrolateral nucleus of the thalamus produced striking improvement in tremor and rigidity. We usually operated on younger patients with predominantly unilateral tremor and rigidity. The tremor frequently ceased as soon as the probe struck the target. It was an exciting era in functional neurosurgery.

Surgical indications abruptly changed a short time after my arrival in Peoria. George Cotzias published a landmark paper in the *New England Journal of Medicine* in 1967, describing the administration of high doses of L-DOPA, with striking improvement in tremor and rigidity. (2) L-DOPA was released by the FDA in 1970, and patients experienced dramatic improvement with this new treatment. Cotzias was awarded the Albert Lasker Award for the work and in 1973, was elected to the US National Academy of Sciences for his contribution to the understanding of dopamine. Few stereotactic procedures were done for a decade.

A few years later the limitations of medical management became apparent and surgery again assumed a role. Dr. Alim Benabid in Grenoble, France made the fundamental discovery that stimulation of the brain at high-frequency perimeters had the same effect as a destructive lesion, but could be reversed by turning off the stimulator. Dr. Benabid's utilization of chronic deep brain stimulation (DBS) to produce the effects previously achieved with destructive brain lesions provided a surgical method that was reversible. Sustained striking improvements in tremor and rigidity are achieved with this intervention with few ensuing complications. The modern era of surgical management of movement disorders began with this discovery. (3) For this major scientific achievement, Dr. Benabid shared the 2014 Lasker-DeBakey Clinical Medical Research Award with Dr. Mahlon DeLong of Emory University.

Essential tremor often produces a tremor in early middle life that sometimes becomes disabling to the point that patients cannot manage their coffee cup. A significant portion of the patients has a familial history. Medical management is often successful, but some patients ultimately are candidates for DBS.

Huntington's disease is an autosomal dominant inherited disorder with a single gene defect that causes degenerative brain changes resulting in movement disorders, cognitive changes and psychiatric disorders. The onset of symptoms is usually in the '30s and '40s, although juvenile Huntington's has an onset before 20 years. Patients have involuntary jerking, writhing movements, and rigidity and muscle contractures with gait and posture impairments. Patients with Huntington's disease require genetic counseling and support systems that may be provided as part of the health care system's overall genetics program, or referral arrangements must be provided. Patients and families have to decide on genetic testing. Some patients elect to forgo testing, unwilling to confront their future, and others seek to address the issue immediately. An established relationship with a psychiatrist experienced in Huntington Disease counseling is valuable and essential in any genetic evaluation.

Patients with dystonia are a separate discrete group spanning a large age spectrum. These patients have involuntary muscle contractions producing slow repetitive movements and abnormal postures. Involvement is sometimes quite limited such as voice and writing dystonia's. Extensive involvement of large muscle groups and paraspinous muscles creates very disabling movements. Dystonias occur in children and adults of all ages and require a physician devoting considerable time to the spectrum of dystonia. These patients often are managed with Botox injections and a physical therapy program, and sometimes extensive functional neurosurgery procedures are helpful.

Most patients with Parkinson's disease are in middle or late life. Tics, dystonia's, and Tourette syndromes are seen in early life, and Huntington's disease and essential tremor can be evident relatively early, requiring a movement disorders center serving the entire age spectrum.

These illnesses are lifelong after onset, and are associated with disability causing change in lifestyle, occupation, and family security. Initially, symptoms and disability are limited and require minimal resources and medical management. Disease progression requires extensive medical management, supportive social systems, physical medicine, and cognitive evaluation. At times, the movement disorders clinic becomes the primary source of care. An integrated healthcare system is obliged to support disabled patients in a large region.

Primary care staff can recognize and initially manage many patients, supported by a background expert system attached to the EHR (Ask Mayo Expert, Up-to-date, etc.). Illness progression requires further neurological consultation. A decision regarding a general neurologist or a movement disorders neurologist in a specialty center is based on the complexity of management needed and the availability of consultants.

The diagnostic and therapeutic expertise of a movement disorders center is essential in the management of patients with complex illness. Patients with moderately extensive disease, without consequential dementia, benefit most from a highly integrated multidisciplinary care model. A health care system may develop this expertise or establish an affiliation with another comprehensive neurological center. The decision is based on the volume of care involved and cost structure.

The INI movement disorders center is staffed by two fellowship-trained specialty neurologists, supported by several APN's, neuropsychology and social work, with physical therapy consultation available. Faculty recruitment will allow further sub-specialization. Development of a gait laboratory, shared with the Cognitive Disorders Center and the Multiple Sclerosis Center will permit quantitation of gait and balance function and support research studies. Since Parkinson's disease patients, late in their course sometimes have significant cognitive disorders, co-location with the Cognitive Disorders Center is valuable. New mobile device apps have potential for transformation, allowing constant monitoring with web-based telemetry. Functional information transmitted to the physician's clinic daily, during trials or adjustment, may diminish need for patient visits and travel.

A functional neurosurgeon, available to provide prompt consultation, is essential in a comprehensive center. At the INI, one of the movement neurologists dedicates 1-2 days per week for intraoperative neuro-physiology during DBS surgery. There is a continued role in programming the deep brain stimulator to achieve optimum improvement. The functional neurosurgery program demands a committed fellowship-trained neurosurgeon devoting one-quarter to one-half time to the program. Maintenance of surgical competence and value entails a volume of 20-40 cases per year. DBS has become a significant factor in the treatment of a portion of patients with Parkinson's disease and essential tremor.

A multi-hospital system, operating in an extended region, is best served by a comprehensive center that supports appropriately distributed outreach clinics staffed by specialty APN's with TeleNeurology from the Comprehensive Center. (4, 5, 6, 7) A comprehensive center provides educational programs for primary care providers, increasing awareness of medical and DBS advances, and prevents potential diagnostic mistakes and therapeutic misadventures. Prompt consultation and intermittent chronic re-evaluation, serving primary care providers, most effectively serves the population health need. A destination center utilizing team care and geographically dispersed outreach clinics provide care promptly while keeping patient and family travel to a minimum.

Support systems are essential for optimum care of patients and families and are difficult to provide over a wide area. Support for informal care providers and empowerment of self-management are essential. Web-based support groups have potential for easing family stress. We have not fully explored the potential of patient specialty web-based support systems for our patients. An e-mail based hot line has been utilized by some systems and now can be utilized in the EPIC-based My-Chart system. (My-Chart is the web-based access that EPIC provides, allowing patients to review information generated by their physician) In a specialty center with a large population base, disseminated physical therapists and social workers provide support with problems of balance, falls, gait, and daily living.

In 1997, the National Institute of Neurological Diseases and Stroke (NINDS) released applications to establish the first Morris K. Udall Centers of Excellence for Parkinson's Disease Research to honor former Congressman Morris Udall of Arizona. There are currently Udall Centers at Emory University, The Feinstein Institute for Medical Research, Johns Hopkins, Mayo Clinic Jacksonville, Northwestern University, University of Miami, University of Michigan, University of Pennsylvania, and the University of Washington. This program funds multidisciplinary Centers of Excellence that can rapidly advance innovative research to improve the understanding and treatment of Parkinson's disease and related disorders.

Udall centers perform state-of-the-art basic, translational, and clinical research on Parkinson's Disease (PD). Underlying neurobiological, and neuropathological mechanisms are studied, and disease-associated genes are identified and characterized. Exploration in novel clinical research involves improved PD models, target identification, and early testing of potential therapeutic strategies. The NINDS provides a base for relationships between multiple centers working in the field. The INI has a responsibility to participate in clinical and translational research in PD. Our current ability to meet that commitment is limited by our inability to recruit movement disorder neurologists.

Multiple Sclerosis

Jacqueline du Pre, a 26-year-old English cellist, was at the height of her career when she found "I simply couldn't feel the strings". She went on sabbatical for a year, returning to music in 1973. A diagnosis of multiple sclerosis was made in October 1973 and by the mid-'70s recurrent multiple sclerosis relapses caused virtual paralysis. Du Pre died at age 42, in 1987. Multiple sclerosis often brings disability and despair, striking at the height of a career.

In the '50s and '60s, neurosurgeons were seeing many of the neurology patients in the United States because of a shortage of neurologists in non-metropolitan areas. I frequently saw patients who were told that their symptoms "might be multiple sclerosis." Younger patients with neurological symptoms were told they had multiple sclerosis (MS), just as older patients were told they had a stroke. Neurological diagnosis was often inaccurate in the era before CT and MRI. MS was an illness without treatment, and this diagnosis immediately created emotional devastation. Without MRI, it was difficult to definitively exclude the diagnosis, and patients entered a prolonged period of fear and apprehension. Such a diagnostic mistake is now fortunately rare, but MS remains a formidable challenge with many treatments and biological markers in development.

Multiple Sclerosis, a poorly understood possibly auto-immune disorder of the nervous system, affects 110-140 people per 100,000 in northern states, and about 200 new cases are diagnosed each week in the US. A clear geographic distribution is evident with more patients in the northern US and northern Europe. Women are twice as likely to be affected as men.

Multiple sclerosis (MS) is categorized into four clinical groups for treatment planning purposes and prognosis:

1. Relapsing-remitting MS characterized by unpredictable

acute attacks or exacerbations. The disease remains stable between attacks. This pattern occurs early in the course of MS patients.

2. Primary progressive MS characterized by gradual steady progression of disability, without obvious relapses and remissions. It occurs in 15 percent of patients and is common in those who develop the disease after forty.

3. Secondary progressive MS can occur after a period of relapsing remitting illness of variable length.

4. Progressive-relapsing MS, the least common form characterized by steady progression in disability with acute attacks that may or may not be followed by some recovery.

Accurate categorization is essential to utilize new treatments and design clinical research trials. At onset, 85 percent of cases are diagnosed with relapsing-remitting MS with 50 percent transitioning, if untreated, to secondary-progressive MS, within a decade of diagnosis. Primary progressive MS occurs in 10 percent of cases, at onset. Most patients are diagnosed at age 20-40. Although a relatively uncommon disease, the illness is a significant cause of disability and cost because onset is at the peak of their career. Recent progress in neuro-immunology has made early diagnosis and treatment essential to prevent and/or prolong the onset of disability.

The illness has a wide symptom spectrum and is included in the differential diagnosis of many nervous system problems. An MS Center has responsibility for early accurate diagnosis, as well as exclusion of MS when erroneously diagnosed. There are ten FDA approved disease-modifying medications: teriflunomide (Aubagio), interferon beta-1a (Avonex), interferon beta-1b (Betaseron), glatiramer acetate (Copaxone), interferon beta-1b (Extavia), fingolimod (Gilenya), mitoxantrone (Novantrone), interferon beta-1a (Rebif), dimethyl fumarate (Tecfidera) and natalizumab (Tysabri). These medications require knowledge and experience in management. A number of active clinical trials will bring possibly 4-5 new drugs in the next several years.

The diagnosis and staging of MS with improved imaging and biomarkers continue to evolve and the differential diagnosis from Neuromyelitis Optica (NMO) and NMO spectrum disorders is important. The most recent modification of the McDonald criteria (diagnostic criteria for MS) in 2017 is applied to those patients presenting with a typical clinically isolated syndrome (CIS) suggestive of MS. (1) Utilization of the latest version of the McDonald criteria with MRI imaging permits earlier and more accurate diagnosis of MS and exclusion of other causes for the clinical syndrome. MRI studies currently are done at 1.5 T and 3.0 T, and some research programs are studying imaging at 7.0 T. Appropriate MRI sequences and interpretation are critical to follow the course of the disease process accurately.

A health care system needs protocols for consistent imaging and interpretation to decrease undesired variability and to facilitate research and quality measures. The INI continues to struggle with this difficult process; some MRI studies remain inadequate for MS study purposes. When MS treatments were ineffective, precision was less crucial. New treatments and clinical trials require patients to have accurate evaluation and treatment. Effective care now has the potential for significantly decreasing the disability experienced by MS patients. Patients should not experience study repetition because the initial study failed to provide information required for participation in a research trial. This represents a formidable responsibility to patients in the most critical years of their lives. Consistent utilization of imaging protocols from the initial MS diagnosis supports optimum care and clinical research. Changes in radiology department processes are required. A patient being evaluated with a possible diagnosis of MS should have imaging satisfactory for MS staging, an MS data base, and participation in clinical trials. A repeated imaging study should only be necessary when dictated by the course of the disease or research protocol.

Specific biomarkers are currently unavailable for MS. Increased immunoglobulin G (IgG) index or the presence of oligoclonal bands identified in the cerebrospinal fluid (CSF) samples support an MS diagnosis. Aquaporin 4 (AQP4) antibody assay assists in the differential diagnostic process of NMO and NMO spectrum. Identification of new diagnostic and staging biomarkers remains an elusive research goal. Much of the diagnosis and clinical classification remains dependent on clinical experience.

Neuro-ophthalmologists have an essential role in the evaluation of visual function in MS patients. High-resolution spectral domain optical coherence tomography (a method permitting measurement of the thickness of the retinal layers) has value in assessing visual involvement. Facilities providing visual evoked potential measurements are a part of a comprehensive destination MS center.

The INI Multiple Sclerosis center participates in multiple clinical trials as the neuro-immunological management of MS evolves. This allows the center to offer the full spectrum of emerging therapies to complex MS patients. Patients who are having clinical difficulty seek out new trials hoping to achieve improvement with the trial medication.

A number of patients are now treated with intravenous Tysarbri (Natalizumab) infusion. This is most comfortably done for the patient within the MS clinic, rather than an infusion center serving multiple other clinical programs. Site selection for MS infusion is a conflict between patient and family emotional comfort and system economic efficiency. Large infusion centers, serving patients with different diseases, have economic advantage, but lack the emotional support of an MS Center. Increasing numbers of oral medications may soon make infusion therapy unnecessary or at least less frequent.

Because MS is a lifelong disease entailing chronic management, the MS neurologist often becomes the patient's primary care physician. A team structure is necessary to care for a large number of patients, many with substantial disability. The specter of an MS diagnosis creates an emotional diagnostic emergency, and the MS neurologist must be available to see new patients in a timely fashion. An experienced MS APN can manage follow up visits with support from social work. Availability of a physical therapist in the clinic is an asset for the management of spasticity and other physical problems that arise. Because of disability limitations, appropriately spaced geographic outreach clinics, staffed by an APN with TeleNeurology expertise, can support the regional responsibility to MS patients. Confidence in team expertise and availability diminishes the fear associated with the unpredictable character of the illness.

Cost structure is a major challenge in MS care. The cost of disease-modifying therapies (DMT) has increased more than general pharmaceutical inflation. First generation DMTs originally costing $8,000 to $11,000, now cost $60,000 annually. Newer drugs cost 25 percent to 60 percent more, and DMT costs in the United States are two to three times higher than in other comparable countries. (2) Development of biosimilar biologics, as medicines come off patent, does have the potential for significant saving, but legislation and supervision for these biologics are more challenging than earlier generic medications.

Congress passed the Biologics Price Competition and Innovation Act (BPCIA) as part of the Affordable Care Act of 2010, providing approval of two types of follow-on biologics: biosimilar, products with no clinically meaningful structural differences from a brand name product, and interchangeable biosimilars that can be safely substituted for the original. (3) The FDA has yet to clarify the level of evidence required for the interchangeable designation, so most products initially approved will be biosimilars. The expected savings will be less than small-molecule generic drugs, because manufacturing processes are complex and there are fewer competitors. Progress is critically important in bringing the benefit of clinical research to MS patients. Patients ecstatic about dramatic new treatments, only to find they are unaffordable, remain a societal challenge.

Lou Gehrig's Disease: Difficult Choices

Upon arrival in Peoria, I had my hair cut in the barber shop just inside the main entrance of Saint Francis Hospital by Tim Jones, a wonderful man in his late fifties much beloved by the hospital staff. He provided haircuts for patients stranded in the hospital for weeks, and physicians and staff swamped with work. Tim had a smile and an encouraging word for everyone and patients isolated in the hospital needed that smile.

One day, Tim asked me to look at his tongue; he was having a little trouble moving food about and saying a few words for several months. I saw tiny, twitching movements under the surface of his tongue on both sides that are called fasciculations. Fasiculations are an indication of illness of the lower motor neuron within the spinal cord or the brain stem, in this case in the lower medulla oblongata. Their presence indicated Tim had an illness of his motor neurons. The most likely diagnosis was amyotrophic lateral sclerosis (ALS), Lou Gehrig's disease.

I invited Tim to my office the following day, and examination revealed some fasiculations in the shoulder muscles in both arms, in addition to the problem with his tongue. This was one of the most challenging office sessions of my career. I discussed his diagnosis and the ominous prognosis of a patient with the disease presenting with signs of brainstem involvement. ALS results in progressive loss of motor function with weakness in the extremities, loss of swallowing, speech, and respiratory function and is often fatal in two to five years. There was no effective treatment that altered the disease.

Tim felt he was in excellent health, relatively young and had extensive plans for the future. He and Ann, his wife, were devastated. I called his family doctor, and we cared for Tim as he steadily worsened. The barbershop closed. Tim succumbed to respiratory complications, within two years. During that period, there were difficult discussions and decisions with Tim and his wife Ann regarding feeding tubes, tracheotomy, and respiratory assistance. Although the spectrum of the disease is extensive, patients ultimately have difficulty with swallowing, coughing, and breathing. As supportive technology has steadily improved, more and more decisions need to be made regarding their use and effect on quality of life.

Neuromuscular Illness

Stephen Hawking, the famous theoretical physicist at the University of Cambridge was diagnosed with amyotrophic lateral sclerosis at 21 and was not expected to see his 25th birthday. Hawking had used a computer system to speak since 1985, and, at 74 years old, was the director of research at the Cambridge Center for Theoretical Cosmology. Stephen Hawking died in March 2018, 55 years after his diagnosis. The course of his illness was very different from that of Tim Jones. This illustrates the striking variation and complexity of this neuromuscular disease and the evolution of care available to patients.

A neuromuscular (NM) center cares for a large group of conditions involving nerve and muscle, some common and some rare. With time and experience, a number of very different and unrelated illnesses have been included in the neuromuscular subspecialty.

Many are disabling chronic illnesses altering the lives of patients and families. The centers usually care for these diseases:

1. Peripheral neuropathies
2. Myasthenia gravis
3. Amyotrophic lateral sclerosis
4. Diseases of muscle.

The NM center requires a multidisciplinary team to provide care for this disparate group of illnesses that have been assembled and assigned to the neuromuscular section in neurology departments.

1. Peripheral neuropathy consultation and management is a significant and growing population health responsibility. Various frequently occurring diabetic mono and peripheral neuropathies are evaluated and managed by the patient's internist. Support by the neuromuscular center is needed for more complex diagnostic challenges and management problems. The NM center becomes a critical member of a team whose role is to develop diagnostic and management paradigms for this vital component of diabetic care.

   Consultation and management of the peripheral neuropathies encountered in oncology centers contribute to the multidisciplinary care of cancer patients. Collaboration with rheumatology is, at times, helpful in the management of the peripheral nerve manifestations of auto-immune diseases such as rheumatoid arthritis. (1) A significant group of elderly patients with peripheral neuropathies without an apparent cause are seen and evaluated as well.

2. Myasthenia gravis and the myasthenia syndromes, illnesses of the neuromuscular junction producing

fluctuating muscular weakness and fatigue, require the multidisciplinary team support of a neuromuscular center. Patients are plagued with weakness and fatigue, and their diagnosis is sometimes delayed to their detriment. Care is primarily outpatient, and occasionally inpatient consultation, is needed in the profoundly increased weakness associated with myasthenic crisis.

3. The NM Center provides diagnosis and management of patients with motor neuron disease (ALS) like Tim Jones. (3) Although uncommon, these illnesses early in their course often mimic other diseases, and the NM Center works with physicians to increase awareness and early diagnosis. Jean-Martin Charcot, the French neurologist at the Salpetriere Hospital in Paris, was the first to develop the relationship of a number of disparate entities into one disorder. The rapid development of genetic analysis now suggests that indeed, there are different genotypic subtypes, and research trials recognize this heterogeneity. (4)

A new organization, Answer ALS, in September 2015, announced a program demonstrating novel approaches to clinical research. Dr. Jeffery Rothstein of Johns Hopkins, Dr. Clive Svendsen of Cedars-Sinai, and Dr. Merit Cudkowicz of the Massachusetts General Hospital are forming a multicenter program to amass extensive data on 1000 ALS patients encompassing clinical, chemical, genetic, protein, historical, and other biological data. They will employ big data techniques utilizing data sets that can only be achieved with such an extended network. This is a dramatic demonstration of a significant trend in research application of new data management abilities.

4. INI NM Center includes a Muscular Dystrophy

Association Clinic providing care for adults and children with a range of muscular dystrophies and metabolic diseases of muscle. Children with muscular dystrophy require diagnosis, physical therapy, and supportive care. The clinic is staffed by fellowship-trained neuromuscular neurologists, physical therapists, nurses, social workers, and at times, orthotic and equipment specialists. A neuropathologist evaluates muscle and nerve biopsy with histology, muscular dystrophy testing, myositis testing, and mitochondrial studies.

Whole-genome and whole-exome sequencing have made it apparent that muscular dystrophy is not just several diseases but a family of more than 50 distinct diseases defined by specific genetic mutations. (2). MD research has expanded in diverse directions, with potential for novel treatments addressing the specific molecular pathology. Gene editing with CRISPR-Cas9 techniques provides hope for a significant alteration in Duchene muscular dystrophy. (5, 6) Many of these strategies are being actively investigated in animal models, and none have reached the level of established clinical management. Identification and repair of specific gene defects remain an elusive goal. This is one of the very active and exciting areas of investigation in the management of genetic illness.

In September 2016, the FDA approved Exondys 51(eteplirsen) for Duchene muscular dystrophy. (7) This drug utilizes exon skipping to partially correct a genetic defect, allowing muscle cells to produce a functional form of dystrophin. This illustrates the complex scientific, cultural and economic issues involved. The clinical trial included only 12 boys, and controls were not involved. The drug is applicable to only about 13% of the patients. Duchene dystrophy affects 9,000-12,000 Americans, almost entirely boys with a genetic mutation causing them not to produce dystrophin necessary for muscle health. The boys typically are in wheelchairs in their teens and die in their late 20s. The cost is estimated to be $300,000 per year for the medication, and there has been heated debate regarding the quality of evidence for effectiveness. The parent group had appreciable influence in the process. This process generated considerable controversy, with some feeling that scientific rigor had been compromised.

Addae Okafor, a seven year-old boy, born in Nigeria, came to the INI Muscular Dystrophy clinic with his father whose English was limited. The family had immigrated to a community in western Illinois. Addae had moderate weakness in his shoulders and hips and the family was concerned that he could not walk well. There was no family history. Addae had an injection a few months earlier, and they attributed the problem to that. The creatine phosphokinase (CPK), a muscle enzyme, was very high, making a diagnosis of Duchene muscular dystrophy likely. Dr. Blume worked with the MD Clinic genetics counselor and Emory University to become involved with a free diagnostic program for Duchene patients. Genetic testing was arranged with the assistance of the MDA, the genetic counselor, translations services, and Emory University. Duchene Muscular Dystrophy (DMD) is entering an era of testing of exon skipping drugs with individual gene therapies for many of the deletions on the dystrophin gene. This Nigerian refugee boy will be able to participate in medication trials for his disease. All of the DMD patients are being genetically tested to facilitate entry in developing trials. A demonstration of precision medicine, and the increasing ease of multicenter cooperation in the care of complex illness.

NM center physicians also provide consultation and electromyography (EMG) and nerve conduction velocity(NCV) studies to assist evaluation of arm and leg neuropathies of undetermined origin, and consult in carpal tunnel and ulnar entrapment syndromes, and lower extremity radiculopathy. Relationships with orthopedic surgery, neurosurgery, and medicine are important. The NM Center must work with each of these groups to develop protocols and guidelines to support appropriate and timely consultation.

EMG is often done in the United States without an associated clinical consultation and has often been utilized inappropriately and without adequate quality mechanisms. Poor quality EMG sometimes leads to diagnostic error and inappropriate treatment and surgery. EMG should be conducted by qualified neurologists or physiatrists, with appropriate consultation and evaluation of the clinical problem. Professional qualification includes certification in EMG and performance of a minimum of 100 studies per year.

Health care systems serving a population base of 1-2 million require 2-3 neuromuscular neurologists and a pediatric neurologist with NM expertise. Like many neurological illnesses associated with disability and mobility limitations, the patients need both the skills of a complex diagnostic center and local support systems. In a geographically dispersed system, the center must provide more convenient local electrophysiology and outreach clinics for these chronic illnesses with disability, optimally utilizing TeleNeurology infrastructure. Subspecialty trained APNs support chronic management of patients, facilitating prompt consultation by NM neurology staff. Physical therapists and social workers familiar with neuromuscular illness enhance the patient's experience.

Neuro-Ophthalmology

Neuro-ophthalmologists evaluate and care for illness affecting the optic nerve, optic pathways and visual cortex, utilizing a number of complex clinical tests. They enter the specialty from ophthalmology and/or neurology and within the US, they represent a small group of sub-specialists They provide critical expertise in the care of stroke, multiple sclerosis, brain and pituitary tumor, and support ophthalmology and general medicine services. The service, while providing substantial outpatient consultation, also contributes to the destination inpatient neurology teaching service. The INI neurology and neurosurgery residency programs benefit from the teaching commitment of neuro-ophthalmology faculty.

Three neuro-ophthalmologists staff INI neuro-ophthalmology assuring consistent availability. They provide consultative services for extraocular movement abnormalities, visual field deficits, a sudden change in visual acuity, orbital mass and pain, pseudotumor, and retinal and optic nerve abnormalities. Technical support for visual fields and fundus photography is necessary for optimum care. The unit is supported by substantial instrumentation: visual field apparatus (Goldman perimeter, Humphrey Visual Field Analyzer, Octopus Visual Field Analyzer), fundus photography, spectral domain OCT, and electroretinography equipment are needed for both inpatient and outpatient consultation.

Because examinations are complex and time-consuming, and specialized instrumentation is required, a neuro-ophthalmology unit presents a funding challenge in neurology departments and health care systems. Unless quite large, a healthcare system needs a relationship with an external neuro-ophthalmology unit to fill this component of their neurological portfolio. The INI has filled that niche for other hospitals in downstate Illinois.

Pediatric Neuroscience

A comprehensive pediatric neuroscience care program is challenging to develop and sustain with the limited US physician workforce. A healthcare system serving a population of 1+ million requires three to five pediatric neurologists to provide the spectrum of complex neurological care for children. Specialized physicians with pediatric expertise provide epilepsy, headache, and neuromuscular care with a seamless transition to adult life. A Pediatric neurology section can reside administratively either in the Pediatric or Neurology Department in a clinic, hospital, or medical school. The administrative structure must foster supportive integration with adult neurology avoiding professional isolation of pediatric neurology.

A long training program and inadequate reimbursement led to an overwhelming shortage of pediatric neurologists in the United States. Recruitment and long-term retention are supported by a critical mass in a pediatric neurology section. The goal must either be the development of a complete pediatric neuroscience program, or a defined relationship with an external center for the spectrum of pediatric neuroscience care. Professional isolation renders a small pediatric neurology unit within a pediatric department unsustainable. An infrastructure, with advanced practice nurses, social workers, and neuropsychologists improves quality and productivity in the care of epilepsy, headache, and learning disorders. As pediatric patients become adolescents and adults, a seamless transition to lifelong neurological care is imperative. Adult subspecialists care for a number of older children with complex problems, achieving a transition supportive of children and parents. The INI supports the work of the University Of Illinois College Of Medicine and Children's Hospital of Illinois building a sustainable pediatric neuroscience program led by Zhao Liu, M.D., Ph.D., a pediatric epileptologist. A relationship with the entire neuroscience faculty remains a critical supporting element as a vigorous pediatric neurology program is built.

Pediatric neurosurgery is provided as an integral part of the INI general neurosurgery program. Cross coverage by general neurosurgery for shunt care provides medium and large healthcare systems with prompt emergency care for children with shunted hydrocephalous and pediatric trauma. A comprehensive program offers craniofacial expertise with pediatric plastic surgery, neuro-oncology, and complex spine deformity and myelodysplasia care. Most US pediatric neurosurgery programs are located in children's hospitals providing complex infrastructure and collaborative pediatric specialists. Health care systems require this expertise in their portfolio and must either develop a comprehensive program or develop a supportive relationship with a referral center.

Peripheral Nerve

The Peripheral Nerve Center is a point of entry for patients with peripheral nerve injury, peripheral neuropathy, and patients who experience various compressive neuropathies. Peripheral nerve injuries, although uncommon, permanently alter the quality of life. These injuries present immediate management challenges, and require well-designed rehabilitation for optimum recovery. (1, 2) Because nerve injuries are infrequent, timely appropriate care from the onset is often unavailable. A recent review of the National Trauma Data Bank (NTDB) found that prevalence of all peripheral nerve injuries (PNI) in adult victims of motor vehicle crashes range from 0.73 to 0.98 percent. (1) Review of the NTDB in children revealed that of 245,470 children with traumatic injuries, 1386 (0.56 percent) had PNI (2). Plexus injuries were sustained in 212 patients and more distal injuries in the upper extremity in 922, and in the lower extremity in 177. Children also have birth-related plexus injuries with an incidence of about 0.1 percent. It is challenging to provide for an infrequently occurring condition requiring complex care.

The care of peripheral nerve injury is evolving rapidly. New methods of nerve transposition and grafting demand a committed neurosurgical and/or plastic surgery staff to achieve state of the art care. A health care system must provide initial evaluation and prompt triage of these relatively rare profoundly disabling injuries.

Large systems will have neurosurgeons or plastic surgeons with the required expertise for complete management. All acute care facilities require protocols for initial evaluation and immediate care, assuring referral to specialized centers. Accurate assessment and appropriate referral avoids lost time and potential increase in avoidable disability.

Sleep Disorders

At 7:20 a.m. December 1, 2013, the Metro-North train derailed near the Spuyten Duyvil Station in the Bronx killing four people. William Rockefeller, the train motorman was believed to be momentarily asleep, when he entered a 30 mph curve at 82 mph. In addition to four deaths, 61 people were injured and damage was estimated at more than $9 million. The National Transit Safety Board, after a lengthy investigation, concluded Rockefeller nodded off because he suffered from sleep apnea. A diagnostic study after the accident, revealed he suffered from obstructive sleep apnea. He had his usual full night's sleep the night before, had not used sedatives, and had prepared carefully for the next day's work. For two years, he had started his shift in the late afternoon. Two weeks before the accident, Rockefeller was switched to a morning shift with a 4 a.m. start time; a change in work schedule possibly exacerbating the sleep disorder. He had a lengthy pristine safety record and no charges were filed. Screening for sleep apnea was not required of railroad motormen, at the time of the accident. The National Transit Safety Board noted that the derailment probably would have been prevented by Positive Train Control system which had not been installed. (1) A mandate for installation December 31, 2015, was earlier extended three years, until 2018.

Sleep disorders are a significant population health problem in the United States, contributing to traffic and workplace accidents and injury, inefficiency, and diminished cardiovascular health. Industrial recognition is improving, but testing in occupations at risk is largely not required. Recognition and identification of the problem by health systems remain an unrealized opportunity.

There is increased public knowledge and recognition of sleep disorder as a cause of ill health. At OSF HealthCare, sleep disorders are managed by sleep neurology and pulmonology medicine. The electrophysiological recording equipment is maintained by staff that manages EEG and the Epilepsy Monitoring Unit (EMU), reducing cost and improving quality. INI sleep neurologists are essential members of the neurology residency faculty.

In most health care systems, home testing is done on 20-25% of patients or less with the remaining sleep studies performed in a sleep center. Improving biometric measurement technology and home testing are decreasing reliance on sleep laboratories. Home testing provides an opportunity to study in an environment that is acceptable to the patient with a substantial decrease in cost. This represents an ongoing technological challenge and opportunity provided by improving telemetry technology. Many more studies are needed, and they will be done at less than the current cost structure, across the United States.

Currently, home testing provides only a portion of the data obtained in a sleep laboratory. Change may be achieved by attacking the problem differently. The questions being readdressed: what data is required to diagnose and treat disorders of sleep? Some work is now being done utilizing patient sound analysis that potentially could obviate the need for EEG data. (2) Because this problem does involve many people and has such a detrimental effect on employment and societal function, there are opportunities for disruptive technological change. The transition from lab to home testing utilizing changing technology is the immediate challenge.

Unable to Walk, then—
To Frankfurt on Lufthansa

D r. Ed Stone called from the OSF Mother House in Germantown Hills. Ed was an internist who cared for nuns in the infirmary at the Mother House, and he was concerned about Sister Mary Clare, a 75-year-old nun who had until recently served multiple nursing administrative roles at Saint Francis Medical Center. Sister joined the Sisters of the Third Order of Saint Francis in Germany as a young woman and trained as a nurse in Peoria. She was anxious to return to productive work-filled days serving the ill, that had filled her adult life. Over six months, Sister's walking had gradually deteriorated. In the preceding three weeks, the process accelerated and her arms were clumsy and weak. That morning, she was unable to get out of bed, and she could no longer manage her breakfast independently. Her rapid loss of spinal cord function concerned Ed. I planned to visit her immediately, after my office session.

Sister was alert and aware of her progressive deterioration. Examination revealed abnormally brisk reflexes in arms and legs, moderate weakness in both arms including the shoulder musculature, and inability to lift either leg against gravity. Sister's great toe went up when the sole of her foot was stroked (Babinski sign). Bilateral ankle clonus (sustained jerking of her ankle when her foot was pushed up) was present indicating spasticity and probable spinal cord compression. Foot position sense was inaccurate. Her ability to feel pinprick was intact in the arms and legs. My examination suggested a problem in the upper cervical spinal cord at the C4 level or above. I discussed this with Sister, and she accepted hospital admission for study.

Cervical spine x-rays revealed only minimal wear and tear changes anticipated in a 75-year-old woman. Her illness antedated

CT and MRI, so the next morning, I did a cervical myelogram, first performing a spinal tap with a Queckenstedt test. This test involved mildly compressing the jugular veins on each side of the neck. If there were no blockage in the spinal canal, the cerebrospinal fluid pressure measured by a manometer attached to the needle demonstrated an increase in pressure transmitted from the head. There was no movement of the fluid in the manometer, indicating a complete block of the spinal canal. I instilled 3cc of Pantopaque, the oil-based contrast material, and removed the needle. When she was tilted head down, the Pantopaque flowed up and stopped at C 3 level with a smooth moon-shaped block in the canal indicating a tumor impinging on the spinal cord. In women, the likely diagnosis was a meningioma, a benign tumor with potentially a good future.

I arranged surgery later that morning. In that era, with diagnosis established with myelography, and a spinal tap below the spinal canal block, delaying surgery was unsafe. The paralysis might become complete. Sister was anesthetized and placed face down on the operating table with her head resting in a large donut headrest, with care to protect her eyes with pads. Modern pin headrests came years later. The surgery involved incising the midline in the back of the neck, spreading the muscles, and removing the lamina (the roof of the spinal canal) at C 2, C 3, C 4 exposing the dural sac containing the spinal cord.

I opened the dura above the tumor which extended from mid-C 2 to Mid-C 3. Fortunately, the tumor was attached to the dura posteriorly. Meningiomas arise from the dura, and cure requires removal of the involved dura. That is difficult to achieve if the attachment is in front of the spinal cord, and easily done if in the back of the spinal canal. I gently separated the tumor from the spinal cord, using loupe magnification and headlight. Tumor removal revealed a deep indentation in the back of the spinal cord at that level flattening the cord. I took a small graft of fascia from the neck to replace the removed dura and closed the wound. Surgery had taken 2 ½ hours and was uneventful. She returned to room 812 on the 800B Neurosurgery unit. Intensive care units were in the future.

The next morning, she could lift her legs a little against gravity, and her feet were moving better. Each day, there were minor improvements in her arms and legs. Ten days later, she was strong enough to return to the infirmary at the Mother House. She progressed rapidly, and within several weeks was walking independently. Several months later, I was making rounds early in the morning at Saint Francis Hospital and met Sister walking down the hall. She was enthusiastic and told me "in two weeks, I fly to Frankfurt on Lufthansa to visit my family".

Year after year, incremental progress in spine care has followed, and complex spinal surgery is now the largest component of the neurosurgery schedule. The INI Spine Institute has a multidisciplinary team offering virtually every technique available in the world to spine patients.

Spine Health

In a year, between 12 and 15 percent of the US population will visit their physician with a complaint of back pain. Neck and low back pain prompt multiple emergency room visits, contribute to lost work days, and cost more than $30 billion in direct care and $14 billion in lost wages annually in the United States. Spine health in an integrated health system assumes a broad spectrum of patient care responsibilities working with primary care providers, urgent care centers and emergency rooms. The spine center must provide prompt same day access. This approach facilitates a rapid return to full activity with less expense created by inappropriate imaging and invasive treatment.

The approach of Virginia Mason Medical Center (VMMC) in

Seattle to same-day access is described in *Transforming Health Care*. (1) The team assigned this challenge decided the elements of quality for the program were:

1. Same-day access
2. Rapid return to function
3. 100 percent patient satisfaction
4. Evidence-based care
5. Affordable cost for providers and employers

A care plan was developed with red flag identification of nerve root compression requiring immediate imaging and spinal surgery consultation. The remaining patients were seen the same day with the initial visit by physical therapists fostering prompt initiation of treatment. In a relatively short time, all patients were seen on the day of presentation. MRI utilization dropped 31 percent after an evidence-based care path required specific indications for ordering the study.

Early implementation of physical therapy decreased the number of visits below national benchmarks. Utilization of a simple exit measure of patient satisfaction assured detection of system malfunction and achieved high levels of satisfaction. Initially, a classic mismatch between financial incentives and clinical efficiency caused a problem. Reduction in unnecessary tests and care led to poor financial results. Adjustments in the payment system, paying for "Spine Health" rather than unnecessary tests and care was needed to support this approach leading to less disability, cost, and rapid return to full activity.

Nationwide, patients with acute low back and neck pain present to their primary care physician office, their chiropractor, an urgent care center or an emergency room. In many areas, because of physician time constraints, patients are sent for MRI imaging before being examined and subsequent decisions are image driven. This approach often results in referral to a neurosurgeon or orthopedic spine surgeon with delay in receiving an appointment and treatment. Increased lost time, delayed treatment, and excessive imaging are factors in the United States which has the highest usage of spinal surgery in the developed world. An optimum program allows prompt clinical evaluation, determination that conservative management can be safely offered without further imaging, and treatment begun. Significant nerve or cord compression causing motor loss or sphincter compromise (red flag) must be excluded at intake.

Several approaches to achieve prompt care have been utilized: Multidisciplinary protocol-driven care initiated by a primary care physician or APN.

1. Initial evaluation by a physical therapist trained in spine health with protocols to identify high-risk patients. (Implemented in Saskatchewan Spine Pathway Clinics and Virginia Mason, Seattle).

2. Internists who have undergone specialized training, essentially becoming "spine-ologists", evaluate and initiate prompt limited conservative treatment in spine and musculoskeletal illness.

The essential elements of a spine health program are:

1. Seen the same day

2. Exclusion of high-risk signs such as saddle anesthesia or drop foot

3. Initiation of immediate limited conservative therapy.

These programs reduce unnecessary MRI imaging, EMG, and epidural steroids. Patients often return to full activity rapidly without orthopedic or neurosurgical consultation. The INI implemented a same day back pain clinic staffed by an experienced

APN with neurosurgical and physiatry consultation availability. This program has been effective in promptly initiating effective treatment.

Ten percent of these patients are expected to have cervical or lumbar disc protrusions, foraminal stenosis or spinal stenosis requiring surgery with or without instrumentation. Primary operations without extensive reconstruction can be done in medium volume centers by neurosurgeons and orthopedic spine surgeons with a quality assessment program. A small portion of these patients requires surgery of greater complexity. An aging population experiences significant disability caused by spinal stenosis and degenerative scoliosis requiring complex reconstructive surgery.

In the United States, substantial change in operative care of spinal disorders has occurred in the past decade. Deyo in 2010, reported the number of Medicare patients receiving complex lumbar spine fusions for spinal stenosis increased from 1.3 persons per 100,000 Medicare-insured persons in 2002 to 19.9 in 2007, a 15 fold increase. (4) At the 2014 meeting of the Congress of Neurological Surgeons, both the President and the Honored Guest raised questions regarding the escalation of utilization of complex spinal instrumentation in the United States. Better recognition of the problem with improved treatment options may be the explanation for increased utilization. Still, a question remains; are we doing too many complex spine operations in the United States?

Symptomatic degenerative scoliosis, primary, and metastatic spine tumors often require complex reconstructive surgery with multidisciplinary expertise and infrastructure. These procedures require multiple level instrumentation. They are done expeditiously with less blood loss and morbidity with intraoperative O-Arm guidance and experienced teams. (O-Arm page 310) INI utilization of O-Arm for multi-level spinal instrumentation has shortened the operative time, decreased blood loss, and decreased early return to surgery.

A spinal oncology program is an element of the comprehensive service. A destination center must serve the small population harboring intramedullary (within the spinal cord) tumors and benign extramedullary (outside of the spinal cord) tumors. A striking improvement in oncology management has changed cancer to a chronic disease, in many patients. Metastatic cancer often involves the spine in these patients, a more common problem than primary spinal cord tumor. Management of complex metastatic spinal tumor benefits from multidisciplinary treatment in a destination center. Management often entails complex instrumentation and additionally may involve radiosurgery or complex fractionated radiation. The health care system must develop a portfolio of services to manage this group of illnesses. (2, 3) Single dose or several fraction spinal radiosurgery is a valuable tool in management of metastatic lesions. Timely application can prevent extensive reconstructive surgery and requires a short visit to a destination center. Experienced interventionalists provide embolization in highly vascular tumors, such as giant cell and metastatic renal cell tumors. A team with extensive tumor experience does resection and spinal stabilization. This portion of the spinal health program can usually only be done in adequate volume in a single center in a health care system.

The INI developed a "Spine School", a one day program to help patients better understand their surgery and recovery experience. The process provides excellent patient preparation for surgery resulting in increased satisfaction, decreased length of stay (LOS), and a rapid return to full activity. The patient knows what they will experience, what is needed the day of discharge, and the exercises and activity they will do in the immediate post-surgery period. Spine School preparation is particularly necessary in patients experiencing complex procedures. A few patients benefit from a short time in a skilled nursing unit or a rehabilitation unit after surgery to achieve a smooth transition and optimum length of hospital stay (LOS).

Intra-operative monitoring is often over-utilized in the United States, and the American Academy of Neurology has outlined specific indications. (1) Monitoring usually is without value in single or two level lumbar disc surgery, only adding cost. Monitoring does contribute to safety in complex surgery within the spinal cord and lengthy reconstructive procedures. Further assessment of the role of intraoperative monitoring continues. Service line protocols foster appropriate utilization of intraoperative monitoring in a multi-hospital system.

Outcome and quality data guide the success of the spine center program. The team must develop and incorporate outcome measures in the electronic health record. Continuous evaluation of individual and team performance is obtained only with timely data extraction. The Quality Outcomes Database (QOD) serves as a national clinical registry for neurosurgical procedures and practice patterns tracking quality of surgical care for common neurosurgical procedures. The QOD lumbar and cervical module developed with the American Association of Neurological Surgeons serve this function. The spine procedures at the INI have been entered in the QOD national data base from the onset of the program, providing a concurrent quality review.

Neurosurgical research has focused on biomechanics and development of complex multi-level instrumented reconstruction. The fundamental reason the spine exhibits extensive degenerative change and deformity in some people, while leaving others virtually unimpaired, remains a neglected research target. An understanding of this biology has potential for positive disruption of the spine industry.

Spine Surgery Joins the Third Revolution: O-Arm Image Guidance

In the past decade, computer image guidance made intracranial surgery more precise and less invasive. Movement between vertebral segments delayed accurate image guidance in spinal surgery because comparable accuracy could not be achieved. Intraoperative images obtained with a portable CT scanner after the patient was anesthetized, and positioned, and immobilized for surgery coupled with the guidance software met the accuracy challenge. The O-Arm with Stealth guidance from Medtronic combined the necessary hardware and software. CT image data is obtained with an image guidance light emitting diode (LED) placed on the spinous process of a vertebra early in the surgical procedure. The CT machine is removed from the surgical field after image acquisition, and the software guidance system is utilized to place the instrumentation in the spine without need for further imaging.

Screws utilized to stabilize the spine are accurately threaded down the pedicle of a vertebrae, a bony structure less than half an inch in diameter that is distorted by the degenerative disease process. If the screw is incorrectly placed, a nerve or the spinal cord may be injured. The guidance allows the operation to move rapidly with less blood loss, and higher accuracy. The screw is placed with guidance comparable to the experience of utilizing GPS to find your way in a complex city. At the end of the procedure, another image set assures that each implant has been accurately placed before the patient leaves the OR. Less than optimum placements can be corrected, avoiding later return to surgery.

Dr. Fassett, Chief of the spine surgery service, led the INI program and continues clinical outcome and cost O-Arm studies. A neurosurgery resident with interest in complex spine surgery assists in this clinical research. This work entails a commitment to improvement of the process, with selection of metrics to determine improvements in quality and cost structure.

Intra-Operative MRI Comes to the INI

Early in the clinical development of MRI, Dr. Peter Black at the Brigham Hospital in Boston in 1995 began preforming operations within the MRI magnet. He utilized a limited number of non-magnetic instruments in a GE "doughnut" magnet. This arrangement provided a narrow space for the surgeon between the two segments of the machine. Dr. Black, thin and small, could fit in the "doughnut". I visited his department in 1996 to determine if early adaptation of this new technology was advisable. Operating within the magnet imposed constraints on the surgical instrumentation. Non-magnetic instruments were clumsy and ill-adapted to the fine dissection required in brain surgery. Positioning surgical assistants was difficult or impossible. I felt that the magnetic field introduced far too many constraints for intracranial surgery. Over time, a consensus developed that surgery should be done outside of the magnet and the patient either moved into an adjacent magnet, or the magnet moved on a rail to the patient to evaluate the progress of the surgery, while maintaining a sterile field. Operating outside the 5 Gauss line of the magnet permitted utilization of the full complement of modern instrumentation and utilization of surgical assistants, resolving my reservations.

The goals of intraoperative MRI were to evaluate the extent of tumor resection before finishing the operation, increase the percentage of tumor removed, diminish damage to the normal brain, and decrease the need for return to OR. Earlier, images after surgery sometimes revealed inadequate removal, necessitating an early return to surgery. Over a decade, technical improvement and experience improved the utility of intraoperative MRI. I continued to waiver; was the improvement in care worth the remarkable cost? After a four year evaluation of evolving technology and fiscal feasibility, OSF HealthCare committed to proceeding with intraoperative MRI in early 2014. The INI began intraoperative MRI in January 2016, with a two-room facility, moving the patient into a 3 Tesla magnet in an adjacent room for imaging as needed. The MRI is used for diagnostic studies when not utilized for surgery, achieving the desired level of utilization of the magnet. Because the MRI is in the operative suite near the recovery room, it is invaluable for pediatric MRI and adults requiring anesthesia.

Initially, this operating room was utilized primarily in surgery for low-grade glioma, where extent of tumor removal is a factor in the length and quality of survival. It is also employed in the removal of pituitary tumors and benign tumors in the base of the skull, assuring the desired extent of tumor resection has been achieved before finishing the operation. Innovative additional uses of this technology are in development at other centers. Placement of a laser fiber in deep brain targets for the destruction of tumor or seizure focus in epilepsy is being performed, avoiding an extensive craniotomy; direct MRI visualization improves control of the treatment process. Intraoperative MRI is being utilized for direct placement of electrodes for deep brain stimulation for Parkinson's disease and essential tremor. In some cases, this permits the utilization of general anesthesia because the placement relies on anatomical rather than physiological data that required the patient to be awake for testing. Among functional neurosurgeons, opinion varies regarding the value of awake physiological testing vs placement based on imaging, a debate not yet resolved.

The INI Brain Tumor Center is the major user of this suite, but intraoperative MRI will have a role in the Epilepsy Center and the Movement Disorder Center, with applications in development.

The $7.5 million expenditure for this two-room unit provides excellent value to our patient population, with use in diagnostic imaging and a host of less invasive, more effectively accomplished surgical procedures. The decision to fund was a culmination of an extensive study of developing technology, a thorough assessment of potential clinical value, and review of a carefully developed business plan. Investment of funds available to improve patient care is an important responsibility never taken lightly.

Bleeding in the Brain, Helicopter Transfer Requested

A call from the PALS operator (the emergency transfer system at Saint Francis Medical Center), at 11:30 p.m., from the emergency room in an OSF hospital in western Illinois, informed me that an 85-year-old man, Oren James, had been found unresponsive on the couch by his wife. She said he had been his usual self when seen only 30 minutes before. She first called her son, who lived a block away, and they had Oren brought to the hospital. His health had been gradually failing, and he and the family had discussed the need for an assisted living facility. Oren was getting quite forgetful, could no longer see to drive, and was on blood thinner for atrial fibrillation, a heart irregularity.

The emergency physician did an immediate CT scan revealing a very large hemorrhage, deep in the left side of Oren's brain. He was drowsy, could not speak and was unable to move his right arm and leg. The emergency room physician requested that we send a helicopter for the 65-mile transfer. The PACS system provides all x-rays taken within OSF HealthCare immediately available for review. The images revealed the massive hemorrhage, deep in the left side of the brain of an anticoagulated patient that would not improve with surgery. His INR (an indicator of the intensity of the blood thinning) was 4.5, quite high, precluding immediate surgery. The outlook was grim, the patient would either not survive this hemorrhage, or remain paralyzed and unable to speak or understand. I indicated that transfer was unwise, neurosurgery was not indicated, and comfort measures were appropriate.

The emergency room physician said Mrs. James and their son insisted on transfer and having "all that can be done". We arranged the requested transfer, the flying weather was perfect, and the transfer was uneventful. Examination on arrival revealed the patient in deep coma, without movement in the right arm and leg. Mrs. James and her son drove, arriving two hours later. I discussed in detail the grim outlook, and they wished comfort measures provided. Oren passed away 36 hours later. We arranged a room for Mrs. James in Family House six blocks from the hospital. She was 83, and although in reasonably good health, found it difficult to be away from home, family, and her dog.

PACS imaging systems and TeleNeurology technology permit evaluation, accurate diagnosis and treatment from a distance. In years past, transfer was not considered in the elderly, resuscitation and respirators were not used, and helicopters were unavailable. Today, all of these technologies are available, and difficult judgments are necessary.

In this new world of virtually unlimited technology, families need help in anticipating what they want as they age and encounter unexpected, and often precipitous illness. It is difficult to first confront these decisions at 1:00 a.m., with much of the family away in another state, and husband or wife in diminished health. Atul Gawande in his excellent recent book *Being Mortal: Medicine and What Matters in the End* addresses this problem. (3) He includes a personal discussion of the long illness of his father and the need for repeated complex, difficult decisions made by the family.

In a society where people routinely live into the late 70s, their physician needs to allocate time to begin this process with the patient and family. Health care teams must consistently make advance directives part of the electronic health record. As we improve, there will be fewer helicopter transfers in the middle of the night, with the later arrival of disoriented, exhausted 83-year-old spouses in strange hospitals. We will achieve a more humane world; it involves identification of the problems, focus, and commitment.

This problem is not new; an original provision in the Medicare legislation compensating physicians for the time to do this work was removed. Legislators associated end-of-life planning with "death panels" and rationing of care. It is neither, rather a first step in helping people deal with technology that has advanced faster than our social infrastructure. (1, 2,). Recently physician reimbursement for end-of-life planning was again included in Medicare regulations. In the United States, fewer than 10% of people 60 years or older have an end-of-life plan in place. Local exceptions exist; 96% of patients who die in La Cross, Wisconsin die with an "advance directive" specifying their decisions about how they would like to die. This was the result of work by Bud Hammes, Ph.D., and the Gunderson Health System over a number of years.

An adequate plan involves the entire family with an attempt at consensus. This allows the spouse and children to better deal with difficult care decisions when emergencies occur. The changed role of the family physician leads to emergency and hospitalist physicians discussing these issues with patients and families to assure patients receive the care they desire. Replication of what was accomplished in a small city in Wisconsin is not only possible, it is imperative, a matter for the urgent agenda in all health care systems.

Chapter 9

The Final Hurrah:
New Challenges
2014-?

You are never too old to set another goal
or to dream a new dream.

— C. S. Lewis

Succession Planning

On my arrival in Peoria in 1961, time seemed unlimited, and I had forever to accomplish my goals. The reality of a finite period was obvious by the '90s. My life was a process of repeatedly leaving positions and readjusting focus. After formation of the Peoria School of Medicine in 1970, we continued as a clinical neuroscience department including neurology and neurosurgery. There had been relatively little precedent for that departmental structure in the United States. Dr. Norman Dott, pioneer neurosurgeon in Edinburgh, was an advocate of this unconventional structure. Dott delivered a convincing lecture at the Congress of Neurological Surgeons on the integration of specialty medicine. Dr. Charles Drake, Chief of Neurosurgery at the University of Western Ontario, developed a clinical neuroscience department that provided the clinical base for striking developments in cerebrovascular care. We utilized this administrative structure for the initial fifteen years in the College of Medicine.

Further development of a diverse multi-specialty neurology department required leadership. Recruitment in neurology proved impossible with our existing clinical neuroscience administrative structure. Most neurologists in the United States trained in a conventional independent neurology department. They were concerned our administrative structure diminished the independence of neurology. I asked the Dean to create a neurology department and change the original neuroscience department to the neurosurgery department. Financial constraints made change difficult, but ultimately a compromise dealt with the financial limitations. We adopted a conventional academic structure in the university and hospital; we established an independent neurology department.

Dr. Jorge Kattah, Vice Chairman of Neurology at Georgetown University, first assumed the role of neurology residency program director and later, in 2000, became the Professor and Head of Neurology at the University of Illinois College of Medicine at Peoria. Dr. Kattah continues to lead a rapidly developing academic neurology department with multiple vigorous subspecialty sections. My administrative role in neurology was officially finished. The first experience with a change in focus and succession planning. Time to let go!

I next retired from the Neurosurgery Headship January 2004 and was awarded Professor Emeritus status by the Board of Trustees October 2004. Dr. Dzung Dinh, Director of the spine service, became Interim Professor and Department Head January 1, 2004, and assumed the Headship January 2005. Dr. Dinh, the fourth resident to finish our neurosurgery program, joined Tulane University in 1991, leading their spine surgery service. He was promoted to Associate Professor and Program Director of their neurosurgery residency. We asked Dzung to assume leadership of the spine section in 1999. Retirement from the Headship was a major life transition. The neurosurgery department was a 365 day per year fixation, for over 30 years. One more step in the "letting go" process, still not easy.

In 2000, I assumed directorship of INI, an administrative role in OSF SFMC. This commitment eased the retirement from the Headship. The decision to develop a system-wide neuroscience service line in 2008 eliminated all concern of inadequate intellectual stimulation. The INI became an all-consuming commitment. After four years, in the early spring 2012, the INI and the OSF neuroscience service line began a strategic review working with Navvis Healthways, a consulting firm headed by Dr. Stuart Baker.

After the first month's work, Dr. Baker invited me to dinner. Stuart told me that the succession planning for the CEO position should start immediately. My reaction was shock; I had assumed that my work would last forever. I was only eighty, a year younger than Rupert Murdock and Warren Buffet and three years younger than T. Boone Pickens! Old friends and colleagues continued to lead major departments; John Jane at UVA, Al Rhoton at the University of Florida, Bob Grossman at Baylor, and Peter Janetta at Allegheny. On further analysis later that evening, I realized that I was functioning in a conventional conservative environment. I was perceived as old; a revelation and an indication I failed to understand the importance of a sound succession plan.

Several days later, I met with Mr. Schoeplein, CEO of OSF HealthCare. We began a formal search with the support of a national search firm. Some excellent internal and external candidates visited over the course of the next year. Candidates brought experience in neurology or neurosurgery; most were not involved in multidisciplinary programs responsible for population health.

Dr. Anthony Avellino, a pediatric neurosurgery professor at the University of Washington, was asked to become CEO of the INI and NSSL and moved from Seattle October 2014. Tony obtained an MBA from George Washington University. He led the Neuroscience Institute at the University of Washington from inception seven years earlier. The experience in Seattle was excellent preparation for the challenge here. Dr. Avellino approached the task with vigor and enthusiasm. He divided the specialty centers into three tiers to provide focus and priority. The first tier included spine, stroke, epilepsy, sleep and multiple sclerosis.

The succession search for the INI leadership was a valuable experience. Over the years, I didn't devote enough time and thought to mentoring, developing staff, and succession planning. Succession planning should begin with the assumption of a new leadership position. One of the leadership tasks is to assure internal candidates have the opportunity to develop appropriate skill sets. Some institutions make leadership appointments for a predetermined period; five, seven or ten years. The initial appointment of the neurosurgery chairman at the University of Toronto is five years with one renewal. The chairman at Mayo Clinic serves for seven years.

Early in my career, I felt a defined term was an unsound policy. From the perspective of 50+ years, I conclude such policy has merit. It encourages the leader to get on with their agenda, realizing time is finite. The defined term is a constant reminder that a successor must be developed. After ten years, few leaders continue to generate original programs and approach each day with originality and enthusiasm. The Mayo Clinic and the University of Toronto are excellent examples of applying a defined period of leadership. Both institutions have had consistent outstanding leadership. If each of my major leadership positions were a defined period, I would have been more effective in succession planning. An important lesson learned late.

In this "After CEO" period, I have an opportunity to follow my interests, working essentially wherever I find interesting challenges. The next pages are a sampler of my idiosyncratic view of the immediate work necessary to improve healthcare. Although some of these interests are limited to the research and education mission of the Illinois Neurological Institute, many represent major challenges in making medical care responsive to American needs.

We enter an era when the tools for change are extraordinary, the need to change is unprecedented, and healthcare is characterized by conservatism and resistance to disruptive change.

Research Director: Research and Publication Infrastructure

After retirement from INI leadership, I talked with Kevin Schoeplein, the CEO of OSF HealthCare System, about staying on as part-time INI Research Director. My goal was a well-developed

INI research infrastructure supporting research and publication by faculty and residents. Accomplishing change in health care delivery and process improvement was an ill-defined second goal. Additionally, I hoped to be a "John Shroyer" mentor to residents and medical students. We had been at the medical school effort for 45 years, and I was acutely aware of the opportunities to be a "Shroyer", which I had missed. In both the neurology and neurosurgery residencies, people with talent and potential were joining the program, and mentoring was needed to assist them to reach their potential.

Training physicians and medical leaders with the new required skill sets is the challenge. Future physicians will measure outcomes, and evaluate and improve processes while leading teams. Leaders need clinical research skills not included in their prior training. Our residents and faculty benefit from an infrastructure supporting clinical and laboratory research and publication of findings. I lacked that exposure in medical school and residency, and failed to independently develop those skills, creating a serious career skill deficiency. Lack of publishing limited early academic opportunities and diminished the quality of our medical student and graduate programs, in a formative period. Correction of this deficit is my immediate priority. An editorial office was created in the Illinois Neurological Institute, to support publication productivity of INI residents and faculty.

Writing and publication are essential for continued accreditation of graduate education programs in medicine. Publication is an element weighted in the reputation of the clinician and institution. Another great value is less appreciated; publication forces precision in clinical work, analysis, and writing. Busy clinicians tend to remember only recent favorable cases and forgo critical analysis of their work. When writing a paper, the clinician must be critical and analytical; the paper will be there forever for the world to critique. It is impossible to develop a strong department without a vigorous program of scientific investigation and publication in high impact journals. Commitment to publication ultimately makes less critical work evident.

Electronic medical records, software, and inexpensive computing power have the potential for dramatic improvement in health care quality and cost. Population health brings responsibility for the health of future patients, demanding a culture change by American physicians. Training and experience have been exclusively concerned with patients currently under care. Rather than complain that patients come too late for care, we will assist in the prevention, early recognition, and treatment of presenting problems. "Big Data" capabilities allow improved identification of risk in the population served, targeting patients for education.

Changes in research funding create new challenges. The National Institutes of Health allocates less money for projects supporting fundamental biological research. This is a substantive threat to career development of young investigators and clinician scientists. The Patient-Centered Outcomes Research Institute (PCORI) funds research studies that examine which health care decisions work best for patients and their families. Although important, this expenditure has less potential for momentous life-changing biological discovery.

A portion of clinical research is supported by large pharmaceutical and medical device companies. Although helpful and important, limitations imposed on scientific publication are sometimes constraining. Unfavorable studies are often not published. Enrollment of patients in an inappropriate fashion for the financial gain of investigators or departments has occurred, and oversight continues to be an essential responsibility for academic departments and institutional review boards. (1) Major private endowments must become a greater factor in research funding. It is far easier to raise money for a name on a physical facility than for sustained research support.

The Role of a Department

After sixty years in varying departmental roles, my view of the opportunities and responsibilities of a department has evolved. Until the recent changes in residency hours, most physicians spent a large part of their lives functioning in their department yet gave little thought to the role of the department in their professional life. The departmental role changes as the medical student evolves to resident, young faculty, and tenured faculty. I have never functioned in or visited a "perfect department". After 30 years as a neurosurgery department head, and another 15 years observing leadership of departments, it is time for introspection. What is the institutional role of a department in a university or hospital?

1. A medical department is a team of people who complement one another compensating for individual inadequacy. The members are aware of their talents and weaknesses and departmental transparency builds supportive relationships.

2. A department, like a University, is eternal and plans talent and infrastructure development for several decades. The department lives beyond the life of current faculty. Long-term vision is required.

3. A department mentors the professional growth of all members.

4. A department develops a robust educational program assuring each student is challenged to their fullest ability and potential. A department assesses the program frequently and strives to attract talented candidates.

5. Departments have a research program that may be extensive, with substantive external funding, or more modest, primarily devoted to outcomes research. Well-designed

research questions and methodology are critical, and a research infrastructure developed. The research program assures graduates leave as questioning scientists, not mere craftsman obsolete with the first disruptive technology advance.

6. In clinical care, the department assures all the resources of the department are employed on behalf of each patient. The faculty know they have the support and resources of the department at all times. Sub-optimal work is unacceptable.

Observation of deficiencies in departmental function in my institution and institutions visited are the basis for this list. Patients have received less than optimum care when talent and facilities for excellent care resided in the parent department. Students, residents, and young faculty have struggled with problems when support was available and unused. Research proposals have failed for lack of critical review by other faculty. These problems are the result of deficiencies in leadership, collegiality, and transparency of department function.

The department is an essential administrative unit, small enough to be agile and responsive yet large enough to harbor expertise needed to accomplish great things. The role of the department head is an awesome responsibility, not a mere honorific. Finally, commitment to the department does not lead to a "silo mentality". On the contrary, the department is responsible for supportive relationships with other departments, thus building complex multidisciplinary treatment and research teams. A strong department is an excellent institutional citizen.

The Illinois Neurological Institute has neurology, neurosurgery, and physical medicine and rehabilitation departments. There are also divisions: neuroradiology, a division of radiology, radiation oncology, and neuropathology, a division of pathology. Sixteen multidisciplinary centers, such as the Brain Tumor Center, benefit by expertise from these departments and divisions. Administrative structure gradually follows function, but historically, there has always been a discouraging lag in development. A vigorous department remains the accountable unit.

The Role of Endowment

Neurology and neurosurgery faculty of our College of Medicine and the INI remain relatively small for the substantial clinical service responsibility. The service commitment impedes full development of academic and research programs. The departments fund most faculty positions with patient care income, limiting resources available for the development of the academic program. Many university neurology departments with similar programs have a much larger faculty partially sustained by endowment. The endowment is a long-term source of strength facilitating the recruitment of outstanding people. While assuring stability, a 4% per year endowment income means a very substantial endowment is required to make a real difference.

While a health care system has an opportunity caring for large numbers of patients with complex problems, it has a responsibility to improve care processes through research and to train future care providers. Clinical and basic science research requires infrastructure and support, and most significant projects need substantial extramural funding, either from the National Institutes of Health or private foundations. These grants are invariably made on the basis of encouraging preliminary data, research infrastructure, and a research team that assures the grantor that success will follow a major commitment.

Modest long-term funding generated by laboratory or center endowment supports this stage, the venture capital stage of the process. If the work is well done and original there is a substantive pay off as in the world of venture capital. A substantial endowment is invaluable in the recruitment of young talented staff that are the critical building blocks of outstanding healthcare institutions. A destination center research program is developed by some faculty who devote 50 to 80 percent of their time to research. Endowment plays a critical role in support of this function until consistent external funding is achieved. Endowment provides assurance of institutional commitment supporting a sustained productive investigational and clinical career. It is critically important in the competitive recruitment of highly qualified faculty.

As a young, inexperienced department head, I knew that I must develop funding for faculty and resident research, but lacked the background and knowledge to design and execute endowment development. My first opportunity presented itself after I operated upon a family member of a Caterpillar executive with bleeding from a giant ophthalmic artery aneurysm. The executive arranged meetings with the Caterpillar Foundation. Over time, a modest plan for our neurosurgery department laboratory was funded with a $200,000 grant, the full amount requested. I failed to provide an extensive long-term developmental plan with far more funding potential. A smaller request for laboratory funding to the Bielfeldt foundation, a private foundation in Peoria, was promptly funded as well. I did not present a ten-year research plan exciting to donors. I had not recruited faculty members with the required research skills to build a program with sustained competitive extramural funding. My need for a coach is evident in retrospect.

Dr. John Van Guilder, Professor and Chairman of Neurosurgery at the University of Iowa, established a professorship for young faculty, an appealing novel approach. An Elwood Professorship in Neurosurgery was created and funded over several years at my retirement from the Headship and activated in 2011.

By and large, in medicine, endowed professorships are awarded to established people, at a point when they have funding, and the endowment is not critical. This professorship was to be awarded for academic promise with an initial term of five years with one potential renewal. It was to be a vehicle for the development of young professors in the tenure track, rather than a reward for established faculty.

We celebrated the appointment of Dr. Andrew Tsung as the first Elwood Assistant Professor on April 26, 2011. Dr. Tsung, a former INI neurosurgical resident, returned from a neurosurgical oncology fellowship at MD Anderson, Houston. An emotional evening at the Country Club of Peoria closed with the unveiling of my portrait painted by Bill Harden, a native Peorian. Dr. Tsung has since established an active brain tumor biology laboratory and a vigorous clinical brain tumor treatment program. The endowment provides a small cushion and is not intended for substantive research support.

Derek Bok in "*Universities in the Marketplace*" (1) and Clark Kerr in "*The Uses of the University*" (2) address the challenges of a research university. A Neurological Institute shares many of these same challenges. Educational and research institutions must endure forever, and endowment provides critical underpinning. Planning and execution have to avoid diversion by short-term,seemingly urgent clinical issues.

Population Health

As the OSF Neuroscience Service Line developed, OSF Health-Care, after study and preparation, asked to be one of the initial 32 Pioneer Accountable Care Organizations. OSF HealthCare committed to being responsible for the health of an identified population, a concept new to physicians. Contributions to the concept of population health developed from the work of the Population

Health Program of the Canadian Institute for Advanced Research and the term has been more frequently used in Canada. (1, 2) Population health has been defined as "the health outcomes of a group of individuals, including the distribution of such outcomes within the group".

Population health is an important paradigm shift, a new way of thinking rather than a new technology. JA Muir Gray points out in an essay that population medicine is not a new specialty, it is a new paradigm that every clinician will sooner or later adopt, with some clinicians being allocated time for working for the whole population. (3) This entails a change in mindset; the clinician is no longer responsible only for those patients presenting to his clinic or hospital, but the entire population his system serves, to the patients they never see, as well as the patients who have consulted or have been referred. Both clinicians and administrators have not thought in those terms. In our previous world, we became responsible when a patient presented himself/herself for care. In population health, we are responsible for preventing illness, early diagnosis, and minimizing cost and effect on the patient's life. This is a new world!

The concept of population health is new and evolving. Many health systems relate this to public health measures, and some specific clinical problems requiring care management such as chronic heart failure and diabetes. Little exploration of population health in neurological care exists, while neurological illnesses are a significant societal stress. Clinicians will be responsible for allocation of resources to maximize value for the population served. They need the right outcomes for the right patients in the right place with the least use of resources and ensure prevention of inequity related to age, gender, race, or social class.

Change in stroke care from concern about "door to needle" time for thrombolysis in a single patient to getting all patients into the system for timely care, and systematic prevention introduces a new set of responsibilities. In epilepsy, specialty centers will help design the initial investigation done by primary care, assuring all patients with a seizure disorder in the population served have optimum seizure control. To be concerned about processes of detection and care for patients yet to be seen requires a dramatic culture change. Health care systems have yet to recognize or quantify the nature and difficulty of this change.

I served on the CMS mandated board of the OSF ACO from inception because I wanted to understand this development. Our data systems were well prepared for supplying the information needed for operating the clinical enterprise, and the medical group met the challenge in the first illnesses identified for measurement. We have yet to accept the population health challenge of epilepsy, dementia, stroke and consistent end of life planning. The first step is acceptance and identification of the new responsibility by the specialty clinicians involved. "Trickle down" is occurring slowly.

Precision Medicine and Genomics

Precision medicine describes new methods that precisely characterize the patient's problem, often with extensive genetic testing and biological markers. It has been further defined as treatments targeted to individual patients by genetic, biomarker, phenotypic, or psychosocial characteristics that distinguish one patient from other patients with similar clinical presentations. (1) President Obama in his 2015 budget message, launched a $215 million precision medicine initiative, with $70 million allocated to the National Cancer Institute (NCI). The NIH received $130 million for development of a voluntary national research cohort of a million or more volunteers to propel our understanding of health and disease. The foundation will be established for a new way of doing research through engaged participants and open responsible data sharing. In summer 2016, the University of Illinois College of Medicine and OSF HealthCare became part of an Illinois research consortium receiving an NIH grant to enroll patients in this initiative.

Francis S. Collins and Harold Varmus of the National Institutes of Health in a *New England Journal of Medicine* essay considered the initiative proposed by President Obama. (2) They highlighted the recent development of large-scale biologic databases (such as the human genome sequence), powerful methods for characterizing patients (proteomics, metabolomics, genomics, cellular assays), and computational tools for analyzing large data sets. These developments set the stage for commitment to a precision medicine program. This differentiates illnesses that previously were considered as the same entity into multiple entities that respond quite differently to a given treatment. Precision medicine will undoubtedly arrive more slowly than anticipated and not live up to the premature hype. Nevertheless, it offers astounding opportunities to improve brain tumor management, provide markers to better categorize degenerative diseases, and to stage multiple sclerosis. Precise characterization of a problem avoids inappropriate treatment. There is immediate hope that cancer patients will no longer endure massive side effects from medicine that is ineffective for their tumor.

The potential for avoidance of risky, potentially damaging, expensive, ineffective treatment is tantalizing. The personal challenge to the primary care physician in handling this deluge of new scientific information is overwhelming, and will only be managed with clinical decision support software utilizing artificial intelligence and machine learning. Medical school and residency programs will include information management in their training programs.

Growing awareness of the vast ecosystem that exists in our bowel, mucosa, and skin, termed our microbiome, adds to the unique characteristics of illness in an individual. (3) This changes our unique immunology, and response to environmental factors, adding complexity to precision medicine.

Already genomic medicine and genetic testing present legal and moral challenges. Companies are providing genetic testing directly to the public based on data of questionable value. Genetic testing sometimes identifies illness with an ominous prognosis, currently untreatable, without consideration of the effect on those tested. This rapidly developing science will demand regulation protecting the public, while not stifling development. These issues are summarized in an essay by Lyman and Moses of the Fred Hutchinson Cancer Research Center. (4) Biomarker science supporting precision medicine is developing rapidly. Annual spending on molecularly targeted oncology treatment exceeds $10 billion, and the FDA in 2015 approved 18 new agents for cancer. Analysis of clinical utility and systems for utilization and reimbursement of these biomarkers must be developed. Biomarker data will have to be incorporated in the electronic health record and medical data collection systems. Biomarker science seems, at this point, to be advancing more rapidly than systems to evaluate, administer, and assure fair utilization across the American population.

Care Paths in Neurological Population Health

Achieving consistent quality care across extensive geography involving multiple locations and clinicians has challenged health care systems from inception. When confronted with 16 subspecialty areas in neurological care, often involving problems that are infrequent and complex, the need for support systems is critical. In neurological care, we have a number of areas where quality metrics remain to be defined. Development of guidelines, protocols, and "Care Paths" has been a response to this clinical problem employed in many systems with imperfect execution. Clinicians have long had an automatic, unfavorable response to "cookbook" medicine or anything that would seem to limit their judgment. System-wide electronic health records offer an opportunity to build safeguards avoiding dangerous or ineffective care.

The Neurological Institute of the Cleveland Clinic, over the past three years, has developed more than twenty care paths. Spine care, stroke, and concussion were the early targets for EHR integration. Care path guides in many systems have reduced variability and unnecessary cost, while improving quality. The Cleveland Clinic experience suggests that the process should include these elements:

1. The care path is evidence driven based on literature, clinical guidelines, and clinical expertise of the representative group involved in the use.

2. Significant pilot testing is achieved before extensive implementation.

3. Consistent updates and modifications are implemented regularly.

4. The technology is effectively embedded in the EMR so that it is an integral element in the workflow.

Ownership by all participants is critical. At the INI, in our first attempt to develop a lumbar pain care path, I failed to involve enough primary care physicians, and those I selected were unaware of the magnitude and importance of the problem. The medical staff was unsure of this encroachment on their autonomy and time. Introduction failed because the initial design lacked the involvement of people providing care; I ignored the process developed at Cleveland. Adequate participation of a large primary care base from the beginning is essential as is sufficient testing before gradually extending implementation. Achieving this participation was difficult because the need and the benefit were not evident to the physicians involved. I did not utilize data demonstrating the pressing need for change in our current methods. Data comparing our utilization of MRI, epidural steroids, and time to return to work, with that of other centers would have made a case for a trial. The testing phase is critical, providing an opportunity to test the concept and make appropriate midstream corrections. Problems in processes can be refined and changed, before implementation involving many patients and clinicians. Actual improvements in quality and cost structure can be accurately quantitated.

This is a process that requires 12-16 months for each major care path to achieve full implementation, involves significant cost and staff time, hence the method should be applied to problems yielding great improvement. The Cleveland Clinic recently published their early results with the Spine Care Path, demonstrating substantial decreases in imaging and epidural injections, with increased use of NSAID's and better documentation of patient education.

Clinical decision support software utilizing natural language processing and machine learning has the potential to make the care path intuitive and less invasive over time. Clinicians aware of the value have to drive this change, it will not be achieved by IT staff.

Natural Language Processing and Machine Learning

Development of the electronic medical record brought potential for great change in the process of evaluating care and performing clinical research. Previously, we extracted information from written or typed charted material recorded mainly in free text.

This was a time consuming, costly process requiring an army of clinical research assistants and others charged with the extraction of this material. With the advent of the electronic record, more information was entered in a structured format. More clicks were required of the clinician, yielding a stereotyped and less informative end product. Information placed in the structured format permitted extraction by computer software, a rapid and inexpensive process. There was a trade-off between the richness of the clinical record associated with extensive free text, and cost of extraction of information for later use.

There is a need to extract information from the record for quality and cost analysis, process improvement, and clinical research. Software applications can be incorporated in clinical decision support, prompting clinicians to supply needed information at the time of entry. A reminder regarding diagnoses, studies to be done, and treatments to be considered decrease mistakes. Each of these changes is enhanced by an ability to utilize free text in a detailed medical record.

Natural language processing (NLP) began in the '50s, a field of computer science involving artificial intelligence and computational linguistics extensively employed in business mainly at a background level. NLP is used in email spam detection, for example, blocking not only specific addresses but searching for content to be blocked. Daily, we are reminded of the potential of this process when we use Google or Amazon. Implementation in health care has been slow, despite having a great unrealized potential for improvement in clinical care.

Beth Israel Deaconess Medical Center in Boston has utilized NLP heavily the past ten years, with successful application in synchronous clinical decision support. Clinicians are prompted to include appropriate clinical data if they have omitted it, to order a test or treatment indicated by a care path, and at times, insurance pre-approval is requested as soon as the clinician has ordered a study.

Natural language processing will assume a significant role in the collation of quality and performance data, allowing prompt correction. It has potential for reducing cost structure in quality management and clinical research. Vendors are developing programs to transition to ICD 10 coding with NLP extraction. This will increase accuracy, decrease omissions, and simplify coding infrastructure required in healthcare systems. Although the complexity and variety of medical care is a challenge; achievements in other industries have created a formidable precedent. (1, 2)

Massive increases in computational power allow utilization of the vast amounts of data available with electronic medical records. Machine learning approaches problems by learning rules from extensive data. Algorithms sift through vast numbers of variables looking for combinations that predict outcomes. Machine learning can encompass enormous numbers of predictors, making analysis previously too complex to be accomplished possible. Obermeyer and Emanuel, in an essay in the *New England Journal of Medicine,* anticipate this will disrupt medicine in three areas. (3) Machine learning will improve the ability to provide prognosis by applying data from large databases, allowing the introduction of many variables. Machine learning has the potential for changing the work of radiologists and anatomical pathologists. Digitized images fed directly into algorithms may generate rapid performance improvement and machine accuracy. Monitoring physiological data has the potential for greatly changing anesthesia and critical care medicine. Machine learning is also believed to have the potential to improve diagnostic accuracy. Anticipating and implementing timely application is an important challenge to health care systems not adequately recognized.

IBM Corporation formed IBM Watson Health, headquartered in Boston, to apply large data to the daily management of medical problems. In late 2014, they released a Point of Care App for multiple sclerosis, providing a comprehensive review of the latest developments in neuro-immunology to the questions arising in the active management of patients with multiple sclerosis.

IBM began working with Memorial Sloan Kettering in oncology utilizing their Watson technology to improve tumor care in 2012. Watson was to incorporate the center's clinical care experience plus the applicable medical literature then apply the acquired extensive knowledge base to individual care. The clinician would continue to make the final judgment regarding diagnosis and treatment, but application of artificial intelligence would greatly augment his/her capability, and decrease errors of omission. In 2018, significant learning has occurred, but the process has proved to be more difficult than anticipated. (4)

Medtronic is working with the Watson Health Cloud to develop highly personalized care for diabetes. The application will receive information from various Medtronic devices including insulin pumps and continuous glucose monitors, providing dynamic personalized diabetic management strategies.

Apple is working to apply cloud services and analytics to its HealthKit and ResearchKit offerings, providing a secure cloud-based system for aggregating massive amounts of patient data. These steps mark the entry of American hardware and software companies into "big data medicine" that will operate at the level of the mobile device, with a potential for rapid change in local medicine.

The challenge is for the leadership of health care systems and academic medical centers to recognize the potential and apply adequate resources in a timely fashion. Their role versus that of proprietary software developers is evolving at this time. Although a health care system need not be a developer, it must be addressing effective utilization of natural language processing, machine learning, and artificial intelligence in its programs.

Cobalt Bomb to Proton Beam

Heidrich family made a significant gift to the Methodist Hospital in Peoria in 1967, allowing them to purchase a "Cobalt Bomb". This was a machine with a large cobalt source for radiation treatment, increasing the ability to deliver a dose of radiation to a tumor. In that era, imaging of the tumor remained relatively poor, hence targeting of the radiation dose was poor. Targeting limitations caused radiation therapy of cancer to be only moderately effective and associated with side effects; "radiation burns". In the ensuing years, imaging of the tumor advanced with CT and MRI, providing an accurate anatomical base for target design. At the same time, linear accelerators were developed that delivered photons in a highly targeted fashion, making radiation a viable part of the armamentarium for cancer. During the same period, as described earlier, we utilized the Gamma Knife to deliver photons from Cobalt in an accurate single dose to targets in the brain.

During this fifty-year period, the staff at Berkeley and Harvard Cyclotrons, on each coast, were exploring the use of protons to treat cancer, utilizing large research accelerators. Protons have a unique property of stopping in the target, the Bragg Peak effect, rather than continuing through the body as photons do. This unique characteristic allows delivery of a higher dose to the cancer with less harm to normal structures beyond the cancer. Until now, these machines were very large, the process was very slow, and a machine cost 135-150 million dollars and required a large, skilled staff.

In the past five years, superconducting synchrocyclotron proton accelerators have been developed. They are compact, allowing creation of a relatively small one-room proton facility at a cost in the $30-40 million range. This has been combined with intensity modulation of a pencil-like radiation beam and precise image guidance, offering the ability to accurately "paint" the imaged cancer with remarkably little radiation to the surrounding tissues. The elusive goal is cure or control of devastating cancers, often located in or near critical structures in the patient's body. This has particular value in treating tumors in children, achieving less radiation dose in adjacent developing normal structures. It also has unique value in treating adult tumors that require high radiation doses for tumor control, but are adjacent to vital structures, such as chordoma in the clivus of the skull base.

Several companies, each with a world-wide presence, are competing to provide single room, moderate cost proton therapy units to care for cancer patients. Proton therapy is becoming available in smaller population centers in the United States. As with all new technology, appropriate utilization will gradually evolve. There is a tendency to utilize the latest technology when it does not offer a therapeutic advance to achieve cost-effective utilization rates.

The challenge is to monitor technology development and select the right technology at the right time. We are engaged in this process at OSF HealthCare, as this is written. While making this decision, we have to be aware of the consistent progress being made in genomic medicine, and the possibility of breakthroughs in targeted chemotherapy and immunotherapy that could replace radiation at some point in the next two decades. Experts are confident that radiation therapy will have a role for the lifespan of the current small proton machines, but the potential remains for biological discoveries making facilities obsolete.

Value in Medicine

There were relatively few tests available for a brain or spine problem in 1961, when I began practice in Peoria. Most tests were inexpensive and medical care was consuming less than 3 percent of the gross national product. Fifty years later, the tests are virtually infinite, and medical care is fast approaching consumption of 20 percent of GDP; suddenly, value in medicine is questioned. The Institute of Medicine, in a recent study, concluded that 30 percent of US healthcare is duplicative or unnecessary. Inappropriate or over-utilized medical tests account for $250 to $300 billion in medical expenses each year. (1) Atul Gawande, in a recent New Yorker essay, noted that the 300 million people in the United States have 15 million nuclear scans, a hundred million CT and MRI scans, and almost ten billion laboratory tests. (2) The fiscal and human cost of unnecessary testing now is a matter for the lay and business press: what is to be done?

The overriding goal is what I term "Straight Arrow diagnosis and treatment"; diagnosis accomplished with minimal, least expensive, least invasive testing followed by appropriate treatment. No detours to the target. In manufacturing, engineers have been charged with making the part as simple and inexpensive as possible, with techniques popularized by Deming. In many medical systems, this view of value is only now being explored. Admittedly, this is a difficult and politically charged process with "rationing, death boards, etc." being used in an inflammatory fashion, when any question is raised about the advisability of a test or treatment. The system of payment for work done, rather than results achieved, has continued to encourage the unlimited use of testing and treatment. The result; higher profits and salaries for providers, the opposite of the incentives imposed in manufacturing.

A transition in payment incentives is occurring in the United States in a slow, fragmented fashion. An adequate response is a management challenge. The Accountable Care Act of 2012 accelerated a beginning trend to "value". This is now a theme for every hospital leader in the United States. Unfortunately, it is not a daily theme in the work of 897,000 active physicians or 200,000 advanced practice nurses and physician assistants. This is where the execution of the needed transformation will occur.

Selecting an unnecessary or inappropriate investigation has multiple consequences in cost, discomfort, and risk for the patient:

1. A simple routine test that is unnecessary incurs only the modest cost of the test. A complete blood count as part of a school physical or hospital admission, without clinical indication, usually only results in the single cost and the rather modest discomfort of the blood draw.

2. A patient presenting with a first focal seizure at age 45 should have an MRI of the brain. He often gets a CT first, which provides much less information, and almost always results in a request for MRI, inserting an unnecessary cost of $800-1500. If the CT fails to reveal a significant lesion, it may stop the investigation and delay diagnosis for 4-18 months or more. CT is much less effective in visualizing gliomas.

3. A patient with a classic benign brain meningioma on MRI may have an interpretation as a possible metastatic tumor by a general radiologist or "night hawk" radiologist not familiar with brain tumor, leading to an extensive investigation for the source of metastatic cancer; an expensive, painful, and time consuming process.

4. Patients may have tests such as prostate-specific antigen (PSA) leading to prostatic biopsy with morbidity that is unnecessary on the basis of current evidence-based recommendations.

Substantive steps are in progress to address this problem. The American College of Physicians has developed a *Choosing Wisely* campaign to address these complex issues. They have developed an extensive system of guidelines to assist appropriate imaging, with a software decision support system that aids execution at the clinic and hospital level. The Neurological Institute of the Cleveland Clinic developed 20 clinical pathways to address these issues and in the past two years have demonstrated performance improvement.

In some systems, a patient with acute lumbar pain after snow shoveling may have an MRI of the lumbar spine done before having an examination by a physician, APN, or physical therapist. This study is unnecessary unless several "red flags" are present indicating significant nerve compression or conservative therapy has failed, and consideration is being given to surgical management. (2)

Opportunity for impressive rapid improvement exists. Health care systems will develop evidence-based care pathways for common problems. Development and utilization of synchronous decision support software will decrease the potential for omission or error. Each care provider and each department has an opportunity to identify opportunities to achieve "Straight Arrow care" by constant Deming-like critical analysis of their experience. The neurosurgery department has a case management conference several days a week; each conference yields a reminder that further attention to test selection is sorely needed.

Several factors contribute to unnecessary testing that are not entirely within the health care provider's control. Fear and cost of litigation are often mentioned as the cause of testing that might be unnecessary. System evidence-based pathways may provide some protection against litigation. Patients often request or demand testing, and avoiding the unnecessary, but requested test requires patient communication. The patient's role in avoidance of unnecessary testing ant treatment is well addressed in Elisabeth Rosenthal's book, *An American Sickness*. (5) Rosenthal addresses the need for informed patients questioning physician advice. A physician pressed for time finds it easier and faster to order an MRI than discuss the reason it is unnecessary. Physicians are graded for patient satisfaction, and refusing a desired test will generate dissatisfaction. Achieving value is not a battle easily won.

Comparative effectiveness research has received increased funding in recent years. We need to train many of our clinicians in research design and develop an infrastructure that makes measurement a part of the care process. A number of measures are available, many incorporating quality of life. Understanding the cost of the entire course of an illness is not fully developed. Downstream costs and savings will be incorporated in the cost analysis: Warfarin in nonvalvular atrial fibrillation is less expensive than aspirin because fewer strokes occur, avoiding the costs associated with the stroke care and the disability. (3) If analysis demonstrates that an intervention is both better and less expensive than an alternative, the intervention dominates. Physicians with new skills are needed to execute this change, and we have not mapped out how this will be accomplished in our medical school and residency programs.

Disruptive change in value may be driven by forces external to the traditional healthcare industry. Warren Buffett has repeatedly stated that "Medical costs are the tapeworm of American economic competitiveness" because we have the highest medical costs in the world, far higher than our competitors. In January 2018, Berkshire Hathaway announced a partnership with JPMorgan Chase and Amazon.com forming a new healthcare company charged with changing the healthcare cost structure. In June 2018, Dr. Atul Gawande was selected to lead the new venture. Dr. Gawande has written extensively about cost and safety in American medicine, and his selection suggests that Buffett-Bezos-Dimon are entertaining strategic changes in care systems, rather than fine-tuning current processes.

Simulation in Education and Care Delivery

William DiSomma's daughter was admitted to Children's Hospital of Illinois after an accident on the family farm, near Canton. Mr. DiSomma was very appreciative of the care provided and sought to contribute to medical care. His experience in the financial world as the founder of Jump Trading gave him an understanding of the value of simulation. This exposure to medical care led to a commitment to improving simulation in medicine by endowing the Jump Trading Simulation and Education Center. OSF HealthCare and the University of Illinois College of Medicine and College of Engineering have been blessed by the Jump Trading endowment to foster simulation and innovation.

In medicine, simulation has been utilized primarily as a training tool and has great potential to change graduate education in neurology and neurosurgery. Simulation offers the opportunity to improve procedural learning with less cost, time, and increased patient safety. In the immediate future, residents will do a new procedure in the operating room only after achieving a required competency in an appropriate simulation.

Simulation offers opportunities in new procedure and treatment design. Fine adjustment of a complex procedure before surgery can avoid complications and morbidity. Multiple procedural variations can be explored pre-operatively, the optimum approach selected, with a decrease in operative time, implant cost, blood loss, and morbidity. This may have immediate application in reconstructive spine surgery requiring complex instrumentation. Maximum benefit from the Jump Trading endowment will require a culture change in the faculty. Separation from their immediate day-to-day clinical concerns is needed to identify and develop the major problems in the delivery of care in neurological illness. In the INI neurosurgery residency program, simulation techniques are in development to foster specific skills prior to application in the operating room.

Patients have extensive experience with computer and information technology and their expectations are changing rapidly. Simulation will bring previously unexperienced clarity in explanation of procedures to patients and families. In the business and commercial world, data can be accessed immediately. Patients are uncomfortable waiting 10 days for a physician's office to call with information. They will not go to the office to accomplish something that in other industries is done online in five minutes. The ability to measure and transmit data wirelessly and transmit digital images with ease requires analysis of conventional office practice. There is a technological base for change in virtually every diagnostic and treatment interaction a patient experiences.

We have to set the cadence of this process and establish priorities for process transformation. The Applied Research for Community Health through Engineering and Simulation (ARCHES) is a collaboration with the College of Engineering University of Illinois at Urbana-Champagne, The College of Medicine, and OSF Health Care System. The opportunity and the challenge is to have every physician, nurse, and care provider ask each day how we can do what we are doing in a simpler, more convenient, less expensive fashion. We have yet to achieve a culture that empowers everyone to generate change. No ideas can be wasted. A "top-down" approach wastes a great deal of creativity. ARCHES provides an opportunity for a fresh look at processes by engineers uninhibited by the "optimum medical approach".

Retail Medicine

Health care initiatives like other industries are cyclic, and "retail medicine" has the attention of the industry. Retail medicine might be viewed as the novel concept of providing the customer with what they want, when they need it, at competitive pricing. Retail medicine is developing rapidly in the United States, performing a "job" for people in an accessible, economical fashion previously unavailable.

CVS developed their retail medicine program providing a limited menu of services, seven days a week, largely without waiting, at a predictable cost. CVS stopped selling cigarettes and characterize themselves as a health care company rather than a drug store chain. This approach has been applied largely to relatively minor acute illness, and to date, has not provided care of neurological disease. The application of mobile technology with the developing "retail approach" has the potential for change managing a broader spectrum of clinical problems.

Amazon acquired PillPack, a company able to provide medication with shipping in 49 states in June 2018. Amazon's involvement in drug delivery with its volume, and international footprint has the potential for significant disruption in medication cost and availability. A secondary effect would be introduction of instability in firms potentially involved in the development of retail medicine.

Walgreens and Walmart have explored this concept as well. The public seeks simplicity, increased availability, and decreased cost. The Illinois Neurological Institute has yet to examine application to neurological illness, but this must come soon. Parents with children who have struck their head, older patients with back pain or dizziness want evaluations on Saturday afternoon, not in 6 weeks at an inconvenient site. What care can benefit from a retail approach? Successful execution may require the introduction of non-health care retail leadership into the development mix. Continuity of care is best served if retail care is developed and delivered as an integral part of the health care system rather in a distinct for-profit entity. Parallel, unrelated systems, have the potential for increased errors in medical care. Will health care systems change rapidly enough to avoid further segmentation of care? The record to date is not encouraging.

Mobile Devices are Changing Medical Care

April 14, 2015, Apple announced ResearchKit, a software framework designed for medical and health research to help physicians and investigators gather data frequently and accurately from research participants using mobile devices. It provides an open source network allowing investigators to build modules supporting their clinical research. Already, academic centers have developed applications that enable patients to be tested several times a day and submit their data with a web-based program.

The rapid proliferation of mobile devices with expanded capabilities is an opportunity and a challenge to clinician's ingenuity. The ability to obtain physical data and transmit that data wirelessly challenges the office care paradigm in yet unimagined ways. Patients who manage a business with a smart phone will find the waiting room intolerable, followed by another wait in the examining room, and a delay at the checkout desk to accomplish something that could be managed with a wireless application.

We are at a decision point that requires a questioning of every patient interaction; can this be accomplished with a mobile device or other technical application? Is this office visit necessary? This is a difficult transition period, with variable acceptance of this technology in the population requiring parallel systems, serving the "new customer and the old customer." Many patients remain uncomfortable with mobile solutions. The division does not relate entirely to age, but to education, and family involvement with technology.

There is a risk in process improvement. Familiar archaic processes continue to be fine-tuned rather than replaced by a markedly different technology. Utilizing a long Six Sigma study to improve a process that needs to be replaced is folly. We are well along the change in managing hypertension, diabetes, and other chronic diseases in some health systems. In the Illinois Neurological Institute, we will evaluate the monitoring and management of movement disorders, cognitive disorder, multiple sclerosis, and epilepsy using mobile applications. Mobile monitoring raises the possibility of obtaining information about a patient's state at numerous times in a day, significantly changing the need for patient visits to an office.

Unique challenges will arise as the "Internet of Things (IoT)" finds use in medicine. Large amounts of data will be processed and converted into useful information. Computer hacking with resulting undesired interventions by third parties is an unanticipated risk. Recent limited hacking in patient monitoring equipment reinforces the need for secure data systems. This will effect how physicians utilize their time, and fixed facility requirements may change dramatically. Like department stores, we may require less office space! Department stores are declaring bankruptcy and closing. Patients may prefer online to the office, mimicking the change in merchandising. Perhaps disruption will be forced on the medical system. We must assist complex patients in a transition to the mobile and web-based world. Already, health care systems have found equipping some patients with iPad or notebook results in decreased cost of care. Virtually every healthcare process deserves questioning re-evaluation and a gadfly to ask the right question. There is a potential for precipitous disruptive change similar to the effect of Amazon on America.

Telemedicine and Neurological Care

Marshall Allen and I were having lunch in Colorado Springs during the annual meeting of the Society of Neurological Surgeons in 1999. As chairman of neurosurgery at the Medical College of Georgia (MCG), Marshall was responsible for providing neurological care to patients over much of rural Georgia. He related an opportunity with AT & T utilizing video to evaluate stroke patients in small towns some distance from Augusta. This was my introduction to the concept of telemedicine as a solution for our distance problems in rural Illinois. Over time, a system incorporating the medical record, images, and video was developed by REACH, a Georgia company that worked with MCG. With REACH, we did an early exploration of the application of telemedicine to acute stroke. Over several years, we explored some technology solutions, and began implementation in thrombolysis decisions in several hospitals in 2013. A profound shortage of neurologists in a medium sized OSF hospital led us to neurology coverage with teleneurology. This application is needed in many of the hospitals served by the INI, but we are limited by availability and willingness of neurologists to staff this service. Development of neuro-hospitalist staffing of inpatient neurology services could be co-developed with TeleNeurology services. A very different role for the general neurologist is being created and will bring change in the neurology residency.

Telemedicine could potentially transform the delivery of medical care in rural America. Although the emphasis has been on the video segment, Telehealth is the provision of healthcare remotely with a variety of telecommunication tools, including telephone, smartphones, and wireless devices, with or without a video connection. Optimum benefit requires recognition of utilization beyond the acute care, remote access solutions that was our initial concern. Telehealth undoubtedly has a role in monitoring of chronic illness. A review by Dorsey and Topol eloquently speaks to three trends leading to wide application of telemedicine. (1)

1. Move from increasing remote access to providing convenience and decreased cost.

2. Move from addressing acute problems to caring for episodic and chronic conditions.

3. Move from hospitals and satellite clinics to home and mobile devices.

The INI is exploring the role of chronic continuing care with regional APN staffed clinics supplemented with Telehealth consultant staffing. First application involves Parkinson and MS patients with limitations in mobility. First based in regional outpatient clinics, there is potential to move into patient homes with further technological development.

Busy patients do not wish to interrupt their day waiting in physicians' offices. Telemedicine may soon be utilized in follow-up and initial visits for specific diagnoses to provide increased convenience and cost reduction.

Significant hurdles and limitations remain to implementation:

1. Reimbursement: Limited and variable throughout the United States. 29 states have some parity legislation in place requiring carriers to pay for some Telehealth service. Medicare only pays in limited rural areas and this has limited Telehealth development. This will change rapidly, but probably at the state level.

2. Clinical care limitations: Physical examination is limited although technological progress is decreasing limitations. Quality of personal interaction is diminished; this may be less important in established patients and younger patients.

3. Legal limitations: State licensure and credentialing limit geographic application. Physician concern regarding liability is a major limiting factor.

4. Social issues: Marked differences in access and familiarity with broadband and telecommunications. Those with the most need may not benefit because of lack of internet access.

We should be asking "is this physical visit necessary" in all patient care. Telehealth, mobile devices, and other technologies may significantly reduce the need for a physical office, clinic, and hospital visits with an associated change in requirements for physical plant. Northern California Permanente found in 2016, they had more virtual visits (email, telephone, and video) than in-person visits. It has been 20 years since my conversation with Marshall Allen, and we are near a tipping point to extensive utilization of "virtual visits" solving access, convenience, and cost problems.

Neurological Portfolio Solutions

Portfolio has been used to describe an artist's work or an investor's collection of stocks and bonds. Complex specialized medical care requires strategic decisions regarding where to provide elements of care, a clinical portfolio. Does a system provide a specialty program in multiple facilities, one facility or is outsourcing the best option? Medical specialty portfolio design, what and where services are provided, is critical for sustainable comprehensive neurological care in a healthcare system. In the past, most hospitals and health care systems prospered despite underutilized and underperforming units. In an era characterized by substantial decreases in reimbursement and margin, a strategy clearly defining focused services and goals is critical to survival and success. (1)

Large systems can offer a comprehensive portfolio but must make disciplined decisions regarding the appropriate facility for a given specialty service. Smaller systems will provide only a portion of the health care portfolio within their facilities. Comprehensive care for their population will entail strategic contracting assuring service, quality, and acceptable cost structure. Each facility can only succeed by performing functions executed with high quality and value.

Portfolio analysis and design begin with a delineation of care needed by the population served. Care needs to be delivered in volume compatible with optimum utilization of physician and staff manpower and facilities. Clinical volume must sustain staff competence at all levels. Competency constraint is generally less understood than cost constraint. Most services have a development period when volume is not self-sustaining. An analysis of the potential for development and a timeline to full development and fiscal and clinical viability is essential.

The model of care alternatives include:

1. Provision of care at multiple sites encompassing the geography served.

2. Provision of care at a single destination anticipating significant patient travel.

3. Offering care by a specific contractual provider at a cost structure advantageous to both, either in the long term, or until the growth of demand makes internal development feasible.

4. Offering care at multiple external providers after assessment of quality and cost structure with specific recommendations and transparent data for patients and health care system physicians.

Factors considered in the analysis:

1. Potential volume based on population incidence data.

2. Cost structure at optimum volume and function.

3. Are physicians and staff available or recruitable to provide the service?

4. Potential of providing destination service for other health systems on a contractual basis achieving target volume.

Optimum portfolio structure is essential to high quality with cost containment. Obstacles to strategic execution:

1. Closure of existing high cost/low volume units is compromised by physician compensation plans and institutional income attribution. As the OSF Neuroscience Service Line developed, many medical practices and hospitals remained reluctant to refer to a specialty center because it resulted in less volume in their facility. Cost and quality data transparency will ultimately drive this transition, but this change is occurring more slowly than in non-medical industries.

2. Patients and families are reluctant to travel for care unless the quality of care is supported by outcomes data. Patients have been unwilling to travel 120 miles for Gamma Knife care or MS disease altering immunotherapy. Focused patient education assists this difficult decision process.

3. A decision to outsource may have unfavorable marketing and image ramifications, even within a healthcare system.

Poor portfolio design leads to providing care in facilities with inadequate volume to sustain staff competency and high cost structure with inconsistent quality. Population health has increased the importance of the portfolio that will be delivered by other providers.

Providing portfolio solutions is an essential function for large specialty centers of the Illinois Neurological Institute. This strategy creates the large patient base required to support multi-disciplinary teams managing complex neurological illness. Execution of a portfolio solution strategy incorporates a value structure, flawless transfer of care, and support of the image of referring health care systems. The referring health care facility must not feel diminished by their referral to a center of excellence. Execution of this strategy is critical for destination centers, yet very difficult in an era of intense competition within large health care systems.

A Return to Where It All Began

I recently reviewed the booklet prepared for my 50th-year class reunion, the Class of 1956 University of Illinois College of Medicine. Our class included three women, one black student, and three Japanese American students in a class of 155. Forward to today, half of the class are women. Black and Hispanic students are still underrepresented but have a significant presence. The medical school class now contains many first and second generation immigrants, a reflection of an exciting change in America and our leading university centers.

Assuming a new role, I interview some students applying for admission to the college of medicine. My experience has been a source of optimism for medicine; the students exhibit surprising diversity. One student grew up in a small village in Nigeria, immigrated to Chicago, attended a junior college, and now is a strong candidate for medical school admission. Others have had outstanding university experience in science, engineering, and liberal arts providing them with unique skills in solving problems in a novel fashion. Most exhibit enthusiasm, idealism, and a desire to better society.

I come away from each interviewing session with one question: What happens during medical school and residency that destroys their originality, creativity, and idealism? We need regular assessment of the undergraduate and graduate program to avoid the injection of cynicism and selfishness that appears with some regularity in the fully trained. To repeat: "Where is John Shroyer?" A faculty that each day reveals the wonder, excitement, and opportunity in medical practice. This is the work of faculty members, curriculum committees, and graduate education review committees in academic medical centers. Naive enthusiasm is a rare commodity and must be nurtured until the end of one's career.

The admissions process favors those who enter university planning to attend medical school and remain focused on that goal throughout their undergraduate experience. In April 2015, a new MCAT examination taking 7 1/2 hours to complete went live. The new Medical College Admissions Test (MCAT) aims to reflect recent changes in science and medicine, removes the writing section, and is scored on a new 528-point scale, with four sections with an individual section score of 132. The new test includes new sections on psychology and sociology and biochemistry. Because students apply to many schools, each college of medicine must cope with thousands of applications, and much of the initial process in most schools is an evaluation of grade point and MCAT scores. The result has been the admission of students that consistently manage the scientific requirements of medical school, but may lack high levels of humanitarian skills.

Despite opening of new allopathic and osteopathic medical schools, a number of US undergraduates fail to find a place in medical school, and elect to attend schools outside of the United States, largely for-profit schools in the Caribbean. These schools provide the first two years on their campus, and arrange clinical clerkships in US hospitals. Thirty-nine of these schools are now operating and enrolling students, three times per year. With increasing US allopathic and osteopathic school enrollment, the off shore medical schools may be unable to place their students in acceptable clinical clerkships. Most of the Caribbean graduates proceed to residency programs in the United States, over half in primary care. The number of graduates achieving certification from the Educational Commission for Foreign Medical Graduates

(ECFMG) increased from 527 in 1995 to 2953 in 2013. This is a significant change in medical manpower in the United States that is still to be critically evaluated. (2)

A number of changes were made in our College of Medicine: students begin seeing patients early in their career, professionalism is discussed and evaluated, and this process continues through residency. "Flipped Classrooms" involve students learning before class online with videos and other tutorial material, followed by an interactive class experience. The old process of endless lectures has disappeared. The first two-year non-clinical period of medical school is shortened to 18 months, allowing earlier entrance to clinical clerkships.

Daily exposure and work with overextended clinicians continue to have a detrimental effect on the educational process. The problem is well identified, a critical first step. (1) I am convinced that medical education is improving, but I am uncertain if we are anticipating the speed of technological change. Since medical school and residency is a seven to twelve-year process, we must prepare incoming students for a technologically different medical world, ten years away. Kaiser Permanente is opening a medical school in Pasadena, California in 2019. Starting with a blank sheet, they have the potential to lead the way in relating medical education to evidence-based team care with utilization of emerging technology.

For the past two decades, medical education has responded to the premise primary care was the overwhelming need in the United States. Primary care remains a major commitment of public medical schools. With changes in the US population, neurological illness is becoming a significant factor in disability and medical cost structure, and we face a growing shortfall in neurological manpower. We need to attract more young physicians to careers in neurological clinical care and research. The INI and the University of Illinois College of Medicine are developing an enriched neuroscience medical school experience. Funding commitment for neurological research experience encourages early exposure to laboratory and clinical research. Mentoring supports and guides the development of a rewarding career in neurological care. This will be my final hurrah.

Let us keep looking, in spite of everything. Let us keep searching. It is indeed the best method of finding, and perhaps thanks to our efforts, the verdict we will give such a patient tomorrow will not be the same we must give this man today.

—Jean-Martin Charcot (1889)

Life is too short to read a bad book

— James Joyce

Acknowledgements

I appreciate the opportunity patients and families have given me to care for them and participate in their lives over a long medical career. In many respects, they have been my teachers in this long evolution of neurological care. Their understanding and support were critical in the early, imperfect days of neurosurgery.

My initial partners in clinical medicine, Drs. Larry Holden, Jack Henderson, Dennis Garwacki, John McLean, and Rich Lee helped through the difficult early days and provided invaluable support during our early stumbling attempts in neurological education. Dr. Holden's unconditional emotional support in the early days made everything seem possible.

My wife Gladys and our children Katherine, Eric, and John provided stability and support with unbelievable patience during the early period of the clinical program and the medical school. Gladys essentially took care of everything "non-medical" in our lives providing a welcoming island of serenity at 1628 Moss Avenue.

Dr. Robert Wright was a true pioneer in the new field of neuro-radiology and catheter cerebral angiography. Bob made a complete abrupt transition to magnetic resonance imaging in 1983 and was a major factor in our clinical success. We worked together each day, and he is very much missed.

The creation of the clinical base of the Illinois Neurological Institute as a seamless provider of the continuum of neurological care was primarily the work of Deborah K. Richardson RN, MSN, NEA-BC. Richardson worked tirelessly to bring together many disparate units into an integrated system for neurological care. Her compensation for my autocratic and insensitive administrative style frequently brought success from potential failure.

The support and advice of the Illinois Neurological Institute Advisory Board was and continues to be a priceless asset. Gerald Shaheen contributed greatly to the formation of the Board and kept it on track. Larry Walden's commitment to providing care to those with multiple sclerosis is sorely needed in all aspects of American healthcare.

Many colleagues and friends assisted in the creation of this book. Critical reading by Dr. William Albers, Dr. Alan Campbell, Byron DeHaan, Marjorie Klise, and K. M. Hashimoto has helped immensely to identify clumsy writing, although I am sure I have evaded their surveillance at times. Deborah Richardson has carefully line edited and reviewed for historical accuracy. Stanca Iacob, MD, PhD, INI research director and medical editor provided invaluable editorial support and review.

Finally, I thank the medical students and neurology and neurosurgery resident physicians who each day continue to bring a sense of wonder and opportunity to my life in my late second career.

End Notes

Introduction

1. Alcon Copisarow. *Unplanned Journey From Moss Side to Eden* Jeremy Mills Publishing Limited ISBN: 978-1-909837-21-8. 2014.

2. Dall TM, Storm MV, Chakrabarti R, et al. Supply and demand analysis of the current and future US neurology workforce, *Neurology* 2013;81:470-478. DOI 10.1212/WNL.0b013e318294b1cf.

3. Nicholl D, Appleton J. Clinical Neurology: why this still matters in the 21st century *J Neurol Neurosurg Psychiatry* 1015; 86:229-233. DOI: 10.1136jnnp-2-13-30688 1.

Chapter 1 Peoria, Early Days: The Family Arrives in Peoria 1932-1952

1. A Timeline of Caterpillar Inc. through the years, *Peoria Journal Star* September 24, 2013.

Chapter 2 Medicine Beginnings 1952-1957

Polio is Conquered

1. Meldrum M. "A calculated risk": the Salk polio vaccine field trials of 1954 *BMJ*. 1998 Oct 31; 317(7167): 1233-1236.

Chapter 3 Beginning a Life in Neuroscience 1957-1961

Spina bifida lifelong care begins

1. Smithells RW, Sheppard S, Schorah CJ, et al. Possible prevention of neural-tube defects by periconceptional vitamin supplementation. *Lancet* 1980; 1:339-340.

2. Czeizel AE, Dudas I. Prevention of the first occurrence of neural-tube defects by periconceptional vitamin supplementation. *N Engl J Med* 1992; 327:1832-1835.

3. Adzick S, Thom E, Spong C, et al. A randomized trial of prenatal versus postnatal repair of myelomeningocele *N Engl J Med* 2011;364:993-1104 DOI: 10.1056/NEJMoa1014379.

Chapter 4 Neurological Center 1961-1970

Neuroradiology

1. Tahir D. Radiology being transformed by cloud, proponents say *Modern Health-Care*, October 4, 2014. http://www.modernhealthcare.com/article/20141004

Intracranial aneurysms

1. McKissock W, Paine K, Walsh L. An Analysis of the Results of Treatment of Ruptured Intracranial Aneurysms Report of 772 Consecutive Cases *J Neurosurg* July 1960: 17, 4, pp762-776.

2. Pool JL. Aneurysms of the anterior communicating artery bifrontal craniotomy and routine use of temporary clips *J Neurosurg* Jan 1961; 18: 98-112.

End Notes

Chapter 5 Medical Education: A New Career 1970-1979

A Medical School

1. *New and Developing Medical Schools*, Michael E. Whitcomb, MD, Josiah Macy, Jr, Foundation October 2009.

Progressive Blindness, Vision Saved

1. Houser OW, Baker HL, Rhoton AL, Okazaki H. Intracranial dural arteriovenous malformations *Radiology* 1972; 105:55-64.

2. Aminoff MJ. Vascular anomalies in the intracranial dura mater *Brain* 1973; 96: 601-612

3. Sundt T M Jr, Piepgras DG. The surgical approach to arteriovenous malformations of the lateral and sigmoid dural sinuses. *J Neurosurgery* 1983; 59:32-39.

Stroke, the End of Therapeutic Nihilism

1. Tissue plasminogen activator for acute ischemic stroke, National Institute of Neurological Disorders and Stroke rt-PA Stroke Study Group. N Engl J Med 1995;333:1581-1587

Farming, My Other Occupation

1. Guyton K, Loomis D, Grosse Y, et al. Carcinogenicity of tetrachlorvinphos, para-thion, malathion, diazinon, and glyphosate *Lancet Oncology* 2015; 16:490-491 DOI: 10.1016/S1470-2025(15)70134-8.

Chapter 6 Neuroscience Residencies 1979-2001

Developing Residencies in Neurology and Neurosurgery

1. Kenneth M. Ludmerer. *Let me Heal: The Opportunity to Preserve Excellence in American Medicine* Oxford University Press 2015.

Botulism Strikes in Peoria, Neurological ICU opens

1. Morbidity and Mortality Weekly (MMWR) CDC, January 20, 1984/33(2);22-3 Foodborne Botulism—Illinois.

Chapter 7 Illinois Neurological Institute 2001-2008

The Illinois Neurological Institute

1. Lochhead RA, Abla AA, et al. A history of the Barrow Neurological Institute *World Neurosurgery* 2010;74(1):71-80. DOI: 10.1016/jj.wneu.2010.07.011.

2. Philippon JH. The development of neurological surgery at the Salpetriere Hospital. *Neurosurgery*. 1996; 38(5):1016-21; discussion 1021-22.

3. Critchley, Macdonald. The beginnings of the National Hospital, Queen Square (1859-1860) *Br. Med J.* 1960; 1(5189):1829-1837.

4. Quest DO, Pool JL. A history of the Neurological Institute of New York and its Department of Neurological Surgery *Neurosurgery*. 1996; 38(6):1232-1236.

5. Feindel W. the Montreal Neurological Institute Historical Vignette *J. Neurosurg* 75:821-822, 1991.

An 80-Hour Work Week: Disruptive Change

1. Bilimoria KY, Chung JW, et al. National Cluster-Randomized Trial of Duty-Hour

354

End Notes

Flexibility in Surgical Training *N Engl J Med*: 2016:374(8):713-727. DOI: 10.1056/ NEJMoa1515724.

2. Birkmeyer JD. Surgical Resident Duty-Hour Rules — Weighing the New Evidence *N Engl J Med* 2016;374(8):783-784. DOI: 10.1056/NEJMe1516572.

Physical Medicine and Rehabilitation

1. Kindrachuk DR, Fourney DR. Spine surgery referrals redirected through a multidisciplinary care pathway: effects of nonsurgeon triage including MRI utilization Presented at the 2013 Joint Spine Section Meeting *J Neurosurgery: Spine* 2014;20(1): 87-92 DOI: 10.3171/2013.10.SPINE13434.

2. Malcolm Gay, *The Brain Electric: the Dramatic High-Tech Race to Merge Minds and Machines*. Farrar, Straus, and Giroux New York 2015 ISBN 978-0-374-13984-1.

Electronic Medical Record

1. Wachter, RM. *The Digital Doctor Hope, Hype, and Harm at the Dawn of Medicine's Computer Age* McGraw Hill, 2015. ISBN 978-0-07-184946-3.

Chapter 8 INI and OSF NS Service Line 2008-2014

Balance

1. Agrawal Y, Carey JP, Della Santina CC, Schubert MC, Minor LB, Disorders of balance and vestibular function in US adults: data from the National Health and Nutrition Examination Survey. *Arch Intern Med.* 2009; 169(10): 938-944.

2. National Institute on Deafness and other Communication Disorders (NIDCD). Strategic plan 9FY 2006-2008.

3. Saber Tehrani AS, Coughlan D, Hsieh YH, Mantokoudis G, Korley FK, Kerber KA, Frick KD, Newman-Toker DE. Rising annual costs of dizziness presentations to U.S. emergency departments. *Acad.Emerg Med.* 2013; 20(7):689-696.

4. Kerber KA, Burke JF, Skolarus LE, Meurer WJ, Callaghan BC, Brown DL, Lisabeth LD, McLaughlin TJ, Fendrick A, Morgenstern LB. Use of BPPV processes in Emergency Department Dizziness Presentations: A Population-Based Study *Otolaryngol Head Neck Surg.* 2013;148(3):425-430. DOI: 10.1177/0194599812471633.

5. Eggers SD, Zee DS. Evaluating the dizzy patient: bedside examination and laboratory assessment of the vestibular system. *Semin Neurol* 2003; 23(1)47-58.

Brain Tumor Care

1. Central Brain Tumor Registry of the United States 2016 CBTRUS Fact Sheet

2. Kahn UA, Bhavsar A, Asif H,Karabatsou K, Leggate JR, Sofat A, Kamaly-Asl ID. Treatment by specialist surgical neuro-oncologists improves survival times for patients with malignant glioma, *J. Neurosurg* 2015;122:297-302. DOI:10 3171/2014 10 JNS 132057.

3. Weller M, Stupp R, Hegi ME, van den Bent M, Tonn JC, Sanson M, Wick W, Reifenberger G. Personalized care in neuro-oncology coming of age: why we need MGMT and 1p/19q testing for malignant glioma patients in clinical practice. *Neuro Oncol* 2012;Suppl 4:iv100-8. DOI:10.1093/neuonc/nos206.

4. Eckel-Passow, JE, Lachance DH, Molinaro AM, Walsh KM, et al. Glioma Groups Based on 1p/19q, IDH, and TERT Promoter Mutations in Tumors *N Eng J Med*

June 10, 2015, 372(26):2499-2508 DOI: 10.1056/NEJMoa1407279.

5. Cancer Genome Atlas Research Network, Comprehensive, Integrative Genomic Analysis of Diffuse Lower-Grade Gliomas *N Engl J Med* June 25, 2015:372(26)2481-2498. DOI: 10.1056/NEJMoa1402121.

6. Louis DN, Perry A, Reifenberger G, et al. The 2016 World Health Organization Classification of Tumors of the Central Nervous System: a summary Acta Neuropathol 2016; 131(6):803-820 DOI: 10.1007/s00401-016-1545-1

Cerebrovascular and Stroke

1. National Institute of Neurological Disorders and Stroke tPA Stroke Study Group. Tissue plasminogen activator for acute ischemic stroke. *N Engl J Med* 1995;333(24):1581-1588. DOI:10.1056/NEJM1995 12143332401.

2. Requirements for Comprehensive Stroke Center Advanced Certification Joint Commission Effective July 1, 2014, issued January 24, 2014.

3. Berkhemer OA, Fransen PS, Beumer D, et al. A randomized trial of intra-arterial treatment for acute ischemic stroke, *N Engl J Med* 2015;372(1):11-20. DOI:10.1056/NEJMoa1411587.

4. Campbell BC., Mitchell PJ, Kleinig TJ, et al. Endovascular therapy for ischemic stroke with perfusion-imaging selection, *N Engl J Med* Feb 11, 2015, DOI:10.1056/NEJMoa1414792.

5. Goyal M, Demchuk AM, Menon BK, et al. Randomized assessment of rapid endovascular treatment of ischemic stroke, *N Engl J Med* 2015;372(11):1009-1018. DOI: 10.1056/NEJMoa1414905.

6. Ebinger M, Kunz A, Wendt M, et al. Effects of golden hour thrombolysis: a prehospital acute neurological treatment and optimization of medical care in stroke (PHANTOM-S) substudy. *JAMA Neurol.* 2015;72(1):25-30. DOI:10.1001/jamaneurol.2014.3188

7. Minimally Invasive Surgery Plus Rt-PA for ICH Evacuation Phase III (MISTIE III) Clinical trials.gov Identifier NCT01827046.

8. Rajan SS, Baraniuk S, Parker S, et al. Implementing a mobile stroke unit program in the United States: why, how, and how much? *JAMA Neurol.* 2015; 72(2):229-234. DOI:10.1001/jamaneurol.2014.3618.

9. Torio CM, Andrews RM. National Inpatient Hospital Costs: the Most Expensive Conditions by Payer, 2011 Statistical Brief #160.Agency for Health Care Research and Quality(US); 2006- 2013 Aug. Healthcare Cost and Utilization Project (HCUP).

10. Fang J, Keenan NL, Ayala C, Dai S, Merritt R, Denny CH. Awareness of stroke warning symptoms-13 states and the District of Columbia, 2005 MMWR.2008;57(18):481-485.

11. American Academy of Neurology, American College of Radiology, National Committee for Quality Assurance, American Medical Association-convened Physician Consortium for Performance Improvement. Stroke and Stroke Rehabilitation Performance Measurement Set. 2012. A comprehensive 75-page document.

12. Disease-Specific Care Certification Program, Comprehensive Stroke Performance Measurement Implementation Guide January 2015 The Joint Commission 206 pages.

End Notes

13. Nogueira RG, Jadhav AP, Haussen DC, et al. Thrombectomy 6 to 24 Hours after Stroke with a Mismatch between Deficit and Infarct *N Engl J Med* 2018;378(1):11-21 DOI:10.1056/NEJMoa1706442

14. 14. Albers GW, Marks MP, Kemp S, et al. Thrombectomy for Stroke at 6 to 16 Hours with Selection by Perfusion Imaging N Engl J Med 2018;378(8):708-18 DOI: 10.1056/NEJMoa1713973

15. 15. Burton T. New Methods Aim to Speed Stroke Care, p A3, *Wall Street Journal* May 15, 2018

Cognitive Disorders

1. Satizabal C, Beiser A, Chouraki V, Chene G, Dufouil C, Seshadri S. Incidence of Dementia over Three Decades in the Framingham Heart Study *N Engl J Med* 2016; 374(6):523-532 DOI: 10.1056/NEJMosa1504327.

2. Jones DS, Greene JA. Is Dementia in Decline? Historical Trends and Future Trajectories *N Engl J Med* 2016; 374(6):507-509 DOI: 10.1056/NEJMp1514434.

3. Langa KM, Larson EB, Crimmins EM, Faul JD, Levine DA, Kabeto MU, Weir DR. A Comparison of the Prevalence of Dementia in the United States in 2000 and 2012 JAMA InternMed.2017;177(1):51-58.DOI:10.1001/jamainternmed.2016.6807.

4. Odenheimer G, Borson S, Sanders AF, et al. Quality improvement in neurology: dementia management quality measures. *Neurology* 2013; 81(17):1545-1549.

Epilepsy

1. Burneo JG, Shariff SZ, Liu K, Leonard S, Saposnik G, Garg AX. Disparities in surgery among patients with intractable epilepsy in a universal health system. *Neurology*2016;86(1):72-78DOI:10.1212/WNL.0000000000002249.

2. Essential services, personnel and facilities in specialized epilepsy centers-Revised 2010 guidelines National Association of Epilepsy Centers Minneapolis, MN U.S.A. Epilepsia 2010;51(11):2322-2333.

3. Kobau R, Zahran H, Grant D, Thurman DJ, Price PH, Zack MM. Prevalence of active epilepsy and health-related quality of life among adults with self-reported epilepsy in California: California Health Interview Survey, 2003. *Epilepsia* 2007; 48(10): 1904-1913.

4. Fountain NB, Van Ness PC, Swain-Eng RJ, et al. Quality improvement in neurology: AAN epilepsy quality measures: Report of the Quality Measurement and Reporting Subcommittee of the American Academy of Neurology. *Neurology* 2011;76(1):94-99.

5. Bergey GK, Morrell MJ, Mizrahi EM, et al. Long-term treatment with responsive brain stimulation in adults with refractory partial seizures *Neurology* 2015; 84(8):810-817.

Headache

1. Loder E, Weizenbaum E, Frishberg B, Silberstein S. The American Headache Society Choosing Wisely Task Force. Choosing wisely in headache medicine: The American Headache Society's list of five things physicians and patients should question. *Headache*. 2013; 53(10):1651-1659.

2. Hawasli AH, Chicoine MR, Dacey RG. Choosing Wisely: a neurosurgical perspective on neuroimaging for headaches, *Neurosurgery* 2015;76(1):1-6.

End Notes

Movement Disorders

1. Michael Kinsley. *Old Age: A Beginner's Guide* Tim Duggan Books 2016 ASIN: B016TG5RGU.

2. Cotzias GC, Van Woert MH, Schiffer LM. Aromatic amino acids and modification of parkinsonism N *Engl J Med* 1967;276(7):374-379 DOI 10.1056/NEMJ196702162760703.

3. Benabid A.L, Pollak P., Louveau A, Henry S, de Rougemont J. Combined (thalmotomy and stimulation) stereotactic surgery of the VIM thalamic nucleus for bilateral Parkinson disease *Appl. Neurophysiol.*1987; 50(1-6):344-346.

4. van der Marck MA, Bloem BR. How to organize multispecialty care for patients with Parkinson's disease. *Parkinsonism Relat Disord* 2014;Suppl:S167-S173.

5. van der Marck MA, Bloem BR, Borm GF, Overeem S, Munneke M, Guttman M. Effectiveness of multidisciplinary care for Parkinson's disease: a randomized, controlled trial. *Mov Disord* 2013:28(5)605-611.

6. van der Marck MA, Munneke M, Mulleners W., Hoogerwaard E, Borm GF, Overeem S, et al. Integrated multidisciplinary care in Parkinson's disease: a non-randomized, controlled trial (IMPACT). *Lancet Neurol* 2013;12(10):947-956.

7. Cheng EM, Tonn S, Swain-Eng R, et al. American Academy of Neurology Parkinson's Disease Measure Development Panel, Quality improvement in neurology: AAN Parkinson disease quality measures: report of the Quality Measurement and Reporting Subcommittee of the American Academy of Neurology. *Neurology* 2010;75(22):2021-2027.

Multiple Sclerosis

1. Thompson AJ, Banwell BL, Barkhoff F, Carroll WM, Coetzee T, Comi G, et al. Diagnosis of multiple sclerosis: 2017 revisions of the McDonald criteria. Lancet Neurology 2018;17(2):162-173 DOI:10.1016/S1474-4422(17)30470-2

2. Hartun D M, Bourdette DN, Ahmed SM, Whitham RH. The cost of multiple sclerosis drugs in the US and the pharmaceutical industry: Too big to fail? *Neurology* 2015; 84(21):2185-2192. DOI: 10.1212/WNL.0000000000001608.

3. Sarpatwari A, Avorn J, Kesselheim AS. Progress and hurdles for follow-on biologics *N Engl J Med* 2015;372(25):2380-2382.DOI: 10.1056/NEJMp1504672.

Neuromuscular

1. England JD, Franklin G, Gjorvad G, et al. Quality improvement in neurology: Distal symmetric polyneuropathy quality measures. *Neurology* 2014; 82(19):1745-1748.

2. Kang PB, Griggs RC. Advances in Muscular Dystrophies, *JAMA Neurol.*2015; 72(7):741-742.DOI:10.1001/jamaneurol.2014.4621.

3. Miller RG, Brooks BR, Swain-Eng RJ, et al. Quality improvement in neurology: amyotrophic lateral sclerosis quality measures: report of the quality measurement and reporting subcommittee of the American Academy of Neurology. *Neurology* 2013; 81(24):2136-2140.

4. Goutman SA, Feldman EL. Clinical Trials of Therapies for Amyotrophic Lateral Sclerosis: One Size Does Not Fit All *JAMA Neurol.*2015; 72(7):743-744. DOI:10.1001/jamaneurol.2014.4275.

5. Calos M. The CRISPR Way to Think about Duchenne's, *N Engl J Med*

2016;374(17):1684-1686 DOI: 10.1056/NEJMcibr.1601383.

6. Wade N. Gene Editing Offers Hope for Treating Duchene Muscular Dystrophy, Studies Find, *The New York Times*, December 31, 2015.

7. Tavernise S. FDA Approves Muscular Dystrophy Drug That Patients Lobbied For *The New York Times*, September 19, 2016

Peripheral Nerve

1. Bekelis K, Missios S, Spinner R. Restraints and peripheral nerve injuries in adult victims of motor vehicle crashes; *J Neurotrauma* 2014;31(12):1077-1082,.

2. Missios S, Bekelis K, Spinner R. Traumatic peripheral nerve injuries in children: epidemiology and socioeconomics *J Neurosurg: Pediatr* 2014; 14(6):688-694.

Sleep

1. Train Engineer in Fatal Derailment is Said to Have Sleep Apnea *The New York Times* April 6, 2014.

2. Doukas C, Petsatodis T, Boukis C, Maglogiannis I. Automated sleep breath disorders detection utilizing patient sound analysis *Biomedical Signal Processing and Control* 2012; 7:256-264 DOI:10.1016/j.bspc.2012.03.002.

Spine

1. Charles Kenney. *Transforming Health Care Virginia Mason Medical Center's Pursuit of the Perfect Patient Experience* CRC Press 2010 pp. 129-148.

2. Nuwer MR, Emerson RG, Galloway G, et al. Evidence-based guideline update: intraoperative spinal monitoring with somatosensory and transcranial electrical motor evoked potentials. American Association of Neuromuscular and Electrodiagnostic Medicine J Clin Neurophysiol 2012;29(1)101-108.

3. Deyo RA, Mirza SK, Martin BI, et al Trends, major medical complications and charges associated with surgery for lumbar spinal stenosis in older adults. *JAMA.* 2010; 303(13):1259-1265.

End of Life

1. Institute of Medicine of the National Academies. *Dying in America: improving quality and honoring individual preferences near the end of life.* National Academy of Sciences Press, 2014.

2. Pizzo PA,Walker DM. Should we practice what we profess? Care near the end of life, *N Engl J Med* Feb 2015;372(7):595-598 DOI: 10.1056/NEJMp1413167.

3. Atul Gawande. *Being Mortal: Medicine and What Matters in the End* Metropolitan Books 2014 ISBN-10: 0805095152

Chapter 9 Final Hurrah: Research Director 2014-?

Research Director

1. Carl Elliott. The University of Minnesota's Medical Research Mess. *The New York Times*, May 26, 2015.

Endowment: What is its role?

1. Derek Bok. Universities in the Marketplace. Princeton University Press 2003 ASIN: 0-691-11412-9.

End Notes

2. Clark Kerr. The Uses of the University. Fifth Edition Harvard University Press, 5th Ed, 2001. ISBN 0-674-00532-5.

Population Health

1. Kindig D, Stoddart G. What is population health? *Am J Public Health* 2003; 93(3): 380-383.
2. Gray JA. The shift to personalized and population medicine, *Lancet* 2013; 382 (9888):200-201.
3. Evans RG, Barer ML, Marmor TR. *Why Are Some People Healthy and Others Not?: The Determinants of Health of Populations.* New York, NY: Aldine de Gruyter; 1994.

Precision Medicine and Genomics

1. Jameson JL, Longo DL. Precision medicine-personalized, problematic, and promising *N Engl J Med* 2015; 372(23):2229-2234. DOI.10.1056/NEJMsb1503104.
2. Collins FS, Varmus H. A new initiative on precision medicine *N Engl J Med* 2015; 372(9):793-795 DOI: 10.1056/NEJMp1500523.
3. Blaser MJ. The microbiome revolution *J Clin Invest* 2014; 124(10):4162-4165 DOI: 10.1172/JCI78366 PMCID: PMC4191014.
4. Lyman GH, Moses HL. *N Engl J Med* 2016; 375:4-6 July 7, 2016 DOI: 10.1056/NEJMp1604033.

Natural Language Processing, Machine Learning

1. Nadkami PM, Ohno-Machado L, Chapman WW. "Natural Language Processing: An Introduction" *J A.M. Med Inform Assoc* 2011:18:544-551. DOI:10.1136/a.m.iajnl-2011-000464.
2. Demner-Fushman D, Chapman W, McDonald C. What can natural language processing do for clinical decision support? *J Biomed Inform* 2009; 42(5):760-772. DOI: 10.1016/j.jbi.2009.08.007.
3. Obermeyer Z, Emanuel EJ. Predicting the Future—Big Data, Machine Learning, and Clinical Medicine *N Engl J Med* 2016;375(13):1216-1219 DOI: 10.1056/NEJMp1606181
4. Hernandez D, Greenwald T. IBM Has a Watson Dilemma *Wall Street Journal* B1 August 11, 2018

Value in Medicine

1. Michelle Andrews. $6.8 Billion Spent Yearly on 12 Unnecessary Tests and Treatments *Kaiser Health News,* October 31, 2011.
2. Atul Gawande. OVERKILL, America's Epidemic of Unnecessary Care, *New Yorker Magazine,* May 11, 2015.
3. Chou R, Qaseem A, Owens DK, et al. Diagnostic imaging for low back pain: advice for high value health care from the American College of Physicians *Ann Intern Med* 2011;154:181-189.
4. Owens DK, Qaseem A, Chou R, et al. High value, cost conscious health care: concepts for clinicians to evaluate the benefits, harms, and costs of medical interventions *Ann Intern Med* 2011; 154(3):174-180.
5. Rosenthal, E. *An American Sickness* ISBN 9781594206757 Penquin Press New York, 2017

End Notes

Care Paths

1. Katzan I, Papesh N. Lessons from the Care Path: Insights on the Neurological Institute's Lead Quality and Value Initiative, *Neuroscience Pathways* 2014, ClevelandClinic.org/neuroscience.
2. Mazanec D. Next Steps along the Spine Care Path: Promising Pilot Results and Fuller Technological Enablement, *Spinal Column* 2014 Cleveland Clinic for Spine Health.

Telemedicine and Neurological Care

1. Dorsey ER, Topol EJ. State of Telehealth *N Engl J Med* 2016; 375(14):154-161/July 14, 2016/DOI: 10.1056/NEJMc1610233.

Neurological Portfolio Creation

1. Porter ME, Lee TH Why strategy matters now *N Engl J Med* 2015;372(18):1681-1684 DOI: 10.1056/NEJMp1502419.

Undergraduate Medical Education

1. Schwartzstein RM. Getting the right medical atudents—nature versus nurture *N Engl J Med* 2015; 372(17):1586-1587 DOI: 10.1056/NEJMp1501440.
2. Eckert NL, vanZanten M. US citizen international medical graduates—a boon for the workforce? *N Engl J Med* 2015; 372(18):1686-1687 DOI: 10.1056/NEJMp1415239.

Glossary

APN Advanced practice nurse. A nurse who has had additional training with a Master's degree in a program specifically designed to develop skills in patient care and management. Originally APN's worked in a role supervised by a managing physician, but in some states now function more independently.

Arteriovenous malformation A collection of abnormal arteries and veins within the brain usually present from birth that predisposes the patient to the risk of bleeding. They often do not cause symptoms until bleeding occurs, although they can be associated with seizures and headache.

Astrocytoma An intrinsic tumor of the brain arising from astrocytes, the cell that forms the supportive structure in the brain. Astrocytomas vary from very slow growing tumors to glioblastoma, the most malignant tumor of the brain in adults.

Beta Amyloid An abnormal protein deposited in the brain felt to be an integral part of Alzheimer's disease.

CME Continuing medical education, programs to provide new information to practicing physicians to maintain their lifelong competence.

Copper chelation Therapies that chemically bind metals to chelating agents to accelerate their removal from the body. Chelation of copper has been utilized in the management of Wilson's disease, an illness affecting the liver and the brain basal ganglia.

Craniopharyngioma A benign tumor that arises in the base of the brain near the pituitary gland. This tumor is common in children and also occurs in adults, essentially in all age groups. Produces visual symptoms by pressure on the optic nerves or chiasm. Often disrupts pituitary gland function and can cause obstruction of cerebrospinal circulation with hydrocephalus and increased intracranial pressure.

Dartmouth Atlas of Health Care Began in 1983, the Dartmouth Atlas indicates variations in health care by geographic area. It uses large claims databases from the Medicare program and other sources to define care Americans receive and correlate expenditures and supply with health outcomes.

Dystonia A neurological movement disorder with sustained twisting and repetitive movements and abnormal postures. It occurs in all age groups.

Endarterectomy A surgical procedure removing atherosclerotic plaque from an artery. The most common site managed by neurosurgery is the carotid bifurcation in mid-neck.

Entrapment syndromes Malfunction of a peripheral nerve caused by compression by adjacent structures. The most common is carpal tunnel syndrome with malfunction of the median nerve caused by compression by the carpal ligament at the wrist level. The ulnar nerve is frequently compressed at the elbow. Many other less common entrapment syndromes occur.

Extrapyramidal signs Abnormal movements seen in Parkinson's disease and dystonia

Fasciculation A brief spontaneous contraction affecting a small number of muscle fibers, often seen as a flickering movement under the skin. Frequently a symptom of motor neuron disease or amyotrophic lateral sclerosis.

Foraminal Stenosis Narrowing of the opening in the spinal canal that is the point of egress of a nerve root.

Globus Pallidus A subcortical structure in the brain, part of the extrapyramidal system involved in the regulation of voluntary movement. Part of the basal ganglia, damage often results in movement disorders.

GME Graduate medical education, specialty education following medical school lasting three to eight years or more. This includes the basic specialty residency, sometimes followed by further sub-specialization in a fellowship lasting one to three years.

Lewy Body Dementia The second most common type of progressive dementia after Alzheimer's disease. Sometimes associated with disturbing visual hallucinations. Protein deposits, Lewy Bodies, are seen in nerve cells in brain regions involved in thinking, memory, and motor control. Visual hallucinations are often an important first symptom.

Metrizamide, a non-ionic contrast agent, injected in the cerebrospinal fluid in myelography to enhance the visualization of structures about the spinal cord. Utilized much less with the improvement of MRI.

Glossary

Molecular Marker In genetics, a molecular marker is a fragment of DNA that is associated with a certain location within the genome. Markers are used extensively in more specific identification of tumors and neurological illness. Markers have great importance in precision medicine.

Myelodysplasia A defect in neural tube development in the formation of the spinal cord, usually presenting as a pouch or defect in the lower spine associated with variable loss of neurological function in the legs, bowel, and bladder.

Neuromyelitis Optica (NMO) An uncommon disease of the central nervous system affecting the optic nerves and spinal cord resulting in visual loss and spinal cord dysfunction

Oligodendroglioma A type of glioma, a brain tumor believed to arise from oligodendrocytes of the brain, occurring primarily in adults and infrequently in children. The classification has been extensively modified in recent years by the introduction of extensive genetic analysis.

Percutaneous angiography, vertebral and carotid visualization of the artery by an injected contrast agent introduced by needle puncture of an artery through the skin, usually followed by the introduction of a small plastic catheter.

Perimesencephalic The space around the mesencephalon or mid-brain

Peripheral Neuropathy Damage to or disease affecting the nerves impairing sensation, movement or glandular function depending on the nerves affected.

PET scan Positron Emission Tomography (PET) scan is an imaging study utilizing radioactive substances called tracers demonstrating function, not achieved with MRI or CT. The tracer is injected intravenously, then the patient is scanned sometime later, and metabolic uptake is demonstrated. This can identify amyloid in Alzheimer's disease. PET is used extensively to demonstrate metabolically active tumors and to study brain circulation.

Physiatrist A medical specialist trained in physical medicine and rehabilitation. Most have one year of internal medicine residency followed by three years of physical medicine and rehabilitation. They have an increasing role in the non-surgical treatment of musculoskeletal illnesses.

Pixilated The individual pixels of a digital image are seen, often degrading the value of the image. A frequent occurrence in the early development of CT and MRI imaging.

Pneumoencephalogram A radiographic study that required replacement of cerebrospinal fluid by air, allowing the ventricles and subarachnoid spaces of the brain to be visualized on x-ray images of the head.

Portfolio This term is used to describe the collection of services a health care facility decides that it can provide with the facilities and professional staff available. This has assumed great importance in a society requiring value. Commonly used to describe an artist's work or a financial collection.

Prion Pathogenic abnormally folded proteins that are transmissible and cause degenerative brain disease. The abnormal folding of prion proteins leads to brain damage and signs and symptoms of disease. These diseases are usually rapidly progressive and fatal. Creutzfeldt Jakob and Variant Creutzfeldt Jakob are the most frequently recognized prion illnesses. Prion was coined by Dr. Stanley B. Prusiner of UCSF in 1982. He received the Nobel Prize in Physiology or Medicine in 1997 for prion research.

Radiculopathy Abnormal function of a nerve root exiting the spine, often causing arm or leg pain

Retrogasserian Neurectomy A brain operation that involved partial cutting of the fifth nerve at the base of the brain to treat severe facial pain, trigeminal neuralgia.

Sagittal Sinus The major midline vein at the top of the brain formed by dura that provides most of the venous drainage of the brain.

SPECT scan Single photon emission computed tomography (SPECT) is a nuclear medicine tomographic technique using gamma rays, providing 3D information. An isotope is injected intravenously, followed by a scan. Unlike MRI or CT, these scans are utilized to demonstrate metabolic function. SPECT is utilized in the evaluation of temporal lobe epilepsy and is less expensive than PET.

Sphenopalatine Ganglion A collection of nerve cells closely associated with the trigeminal nerve that is felt to have a role in cluster headache and migraine.

Stereotactic A minimally invasive method of approaching lesions in the brain utilizing 3D coordinate systems to reach small targets. This has been greatly enhanced with improvements in image visualization of targets and computer power.

Sub intimal injection Refers to the injection of materials between the intima and muscular layer of the artery, often with impairment of blood flow. A frequent complication in early angiography

Sub-Cortical parafascicular surgery A technique to stereotactically pass between major white fiber pathways in the brain to access a lesion avoiding injury to essential brain pathways.

Tangent Screen A black screen used in testing the fields of vision.

Thalamus a large dual lobed mass of grey matter in the basal ganglia involved in sensory perception and regulation of motor function. It is often a target for placement of deep brain stimulation in Parkinson's disease.

Tissue Plasminogen Activator tPA A protein involved in the destruction of blood clots. It facilitates the conversion of plasminogen to plasmin, the major enzyme responsible for dissolving clot. Used as a treatment in acute stroke. It is manufactured using recombinant biotechnology techniques.

Tourette syndrome A neurological disorder characterized by repetitive stereotyped involuntary motor movements and vocalizations called tics. Often first manifested in children between age 3 and 9.

Transsphenoidal Describes an approach to the pituitary gland and other structures in the base of the brain via the nose and the sphenoid sinus. Although a very old procedure, it became useful with the advent of the surgical microscope, endoscope, and computer image guidance

Tysabri infusion A monoclonal antibody that affects the body's immune system used in the treatment of relapsing forms of multiple sclerosis. It must be administered intravenously rather than orally.

Ventriculogram An opening is made through the skull, a needle introduced in the ventricle and the ventricular fluid replaced with air, allowing x-ray visualization of the ventricles and providing localization information regarding brain tumors and other masses in the brain. Rarely done with the advent of CT and MRI imaging of the brain. Developed by Walter Dandy at Johns Hopkins Hospital.

Ventriculostomy Placement of a small tube into the lateral ventricle of the brain through a drill opening in the skull allowing drainage of ventricular fluid. Used to decrease elevated intracranial pressure and to monitor pressure.

Vertigo The sensation that a person or objects about them are moving when they are not. Often associated with nausea and vomiting and difficulty walking. Distinguished from a sense of imbalance or unsteadiness.

Vestibular Schwannoma A benign tumor arising from the covering of the vestibular nerve as it passes from the brain into the middle ear. Often presents with ringing in the ear or decreased hearing. Treated by open microsurgery or radiosurgery, Gamma Knife, CyberKnife, or other radiosurgery devices